Veterinary Drug Handbook

Client Information Edition

Gigi Davidson

Donald C. Plumb

DISTRIBUTED BY

Blackwell Publishing

Worldwide Print Distribution by:
  Blackwell Publishing Professional
  2121 State Avenue
  Ames, IA 50014-8300
  (800)-862-6657

PharmaVet Publishing
Stockholm, Wisconsin

Printed in the United States of America

ISBN: 0-8138-1783-8

Last digit is the print number 9 8 7 6 5 4 3 2

This edition is dedicated to all my Muses, two-legged and four, blood kin or soulmate kin.
With love and gratitude
Gigi Davidson

* * *

Dedicated to people everywhere working to improve the lives of animals
Donald C Plumb

About the Authors:

Gigi Davidson is the Director of Clinical Pharmacy Services at the North Carolina State University, College of Veterinary Medicine where she has practiced veterinary pharmacy exclusively since 1983. She is a Diplomate of the American College of Veterinary Hospital Pharmacists and spends her days providing clinical pharmacy service, mentoring veterinary and pharmacy students, and conducting drug-related clinical research in the many veterinary species. Her passion is the safe and effective use of drugs in animal species.

Donald C. Plumb is the Director of Pharmacy Services at the Veterinary Teaching Hospital, College of Veterinary Medicine, University of Minnesota where he has practiced veterinary pharmacy for over 20 years. He is the author of the *Veterinary Drug Handbook*, now in its 4th edition.

Preface

The goal of the *Veterinary Drug Handbook: Client Information Edition* is to help veterinarians and pharmacists bridge the drug information gap between themselves and the people (clients; owners) who are treating their animals. Several studies have demonstrated that people receiving verbal information from health professionals retain very little of that information once they leave the premises of their health provider. We hope that this information will supplement the actual care provided and help in the task at hand, namely to improve the health of animals. We have included drugs that are commonly prescribed by small animal and equine practitioners, both those that are veterinary and "human" labeled medications. We have also attempted to provide this information in a format that can be understood by any reader. The information presented in these monographs will, hopefully, enable the animal caregiver to be better informed about the medication in question and to work with their veterinarian and pharmacist on the journey to positive therapeutic outcomes.

Gigi Davidson & Donald Plumb
November 2002

For more information, including

- Errata and updates for this edition
- Ordering information for this and other versions of the *Veterinary Drug Handbook*
- Links to other veterinary drug web sites
- To make suggestions for improving future editions of this Handbook,

visit the *Veterinary Drug Handbook* web site at:

www.vetdruginfo.com

Caution!

While a sincere effort has been expounded to assure that the information included in this book is correct, errors or omissions may occur and it is suggested that the reader refer to the original approved labeling information of the product for additional information.

DISCLAIMER

The authors/publisher/distributor assume no responsibility for and make no warranty with respect to results that may be obtained from the uses, procedures, or dosages listed, and do not necessarily endorse such uses, procedures, or dosages. The authors/publisher shall not be liable to any person whatsoever for any damages, or equivalencies, or by reason of any misstatement or error, negligent or otherwise obtained in this work. Should the purchaser not wish to be bound by the above, he/she may return the book to the distributor for a full refund.

Table of Contents

Systemic Medications

Acetaminophen 1
Acetazolamide 2
Albuterol 4
Allopurinol 5
Altrenogest 6
Aminocaproic Acid 7
Aminophylline 8
Amitriptyline 9
Amlodipine 10
Ammonium Chloride 11
Amoxicillin 12
Amoxicillin/Clavulanate 13
Ascorbic Acid 14
Aspirin 15
Atenolol 16
Azathioprine 17
Baclofen 18
Benazepril 19
Bethanechol 20
Bisacodyl 21
Bismuth Subsalicylate 22
Bromide, Potassium or Sodium 23
Bromocriptine 24
Buprenorphine 25
Buspirone 26
Butorphanol Tartrate 27
Captopril 28
Carnitine 29
Carprofen 30
Cefadroxil 31
Cefixime 32
Cephalexin 33
Chlorambucil 34
Chloramphenicol 35
Chlorpheniramine 36
Chlorpromazine 37
Cimetidine 38
Cisapride 39
Clemastine 40
Clenbuterol 41
Clindamycin 42
Clomipramine 43
Codeine 44
Cyclophosphamide 45

Cyclosporine 46
Cyproheptadine 47
Dalteparin 48
Deracoxib 49
Desmopressin 50
Diazepam 51
Diazoxide 52
Diethylstilbesterol 53
Digoxin 54
Diltiazem 55
Diphenhydramine 56
Doxepin 57
Doxycycline 58
Enalapril 59
Enrofloxacin 60
Erythromycin 61
Etodolac 62
Famotidine 63
Fenbendazole 64
Fentanyl 65
Fluconazole 66
Fludrocortisone 67
Flunixin 68
Fluoxetine 69
Furosemide 70
Glipizide 71
Griseofulvin 72
Hydralazine 73
Hydrocodone 74
Hydroxyzine 75
Imipramine 76
Insulin 77
Interferon 79
Itraconazole 80
Ivermectin 81
Ketoconazole 83
Ketoprofen 85
Lactulose 86
Levothyroxine 87
Lincomycin 88
Liothyronine 89
Lufenuron 90
Marbofloxacin 91
Meloxicam 92

Methimazole...............................93
Methocarbamol...........................94
Methylprednisolone 95
Metoclopramide 97
Metronidazole 98
Milbemycin.................................99
Misoprostol................................100
Mitotane 101
Morphine Sulfate 103
Neomycin Sulfate 104
Omeprazole...............................105
Ondansetron 106
Orbifloxacin 107
Oxazepam 108
Oxybutynin 109
Pancrelipase..............................110
Paroxetine 111
Pentoxifylline.............................112
Pergolide...................................113
Phenobarbital............................114
Phenoxybenzamine....................115
Phenylbutazone.........................116
Phenylpropanolamine.................118
Phytonadione (Vitamin K1) 119
Piperazine 120
Piroxicam 121
Praziquantel 122
Prednisone, Prednisolone 123
Propantheline Bromide 125
Propranolol 126
Pyrantel Pamoate 127
Pyridostigmine 128
Ranitidine 129
Rifampin.....................................130
Selegilene 131
Sotalol 132
Spironolactone 133
Stanozolol 134
Sucralfate 135
Sulfasalazine 136
Taurine 137
Terbutaline................................138
Tetracycline 139
Theophylline 140
Trimeprazine with Prednisolone 141

Trimethoprim with Sulfadiazine
     or Sulfamethoxazole 142
Tylosin 144
Ursodiol.....................................145
Vitamin E 146
Warfarin 147

Ophthalmic Medications
Aminoglycosides........................148
Atropine Sulfate 149
Chloramphenicol........................150
Corticosteroids...........................151
Cyclosporine..............................152
Dorzolamide 153
Flurbiprofen 154
Idoxuridine.................................155
Itraconazole in DMSO................156
Ketorolac 157
Latanaprost 158
Miconazole 159
Natamycin 160
Oxytetracycline 161
Fluroquinolones 162
Timolol 163
Trifluridine 164
Triple Antibiotic with Steroids 165
Triple Antibiotics........................166
Tropicamide...............................167

Miscellaneous
Applying Transdermal Medications
     to Cats..................................168
Giving Your Cat Oral Medications .169
Giving Your Dog Oral Medications 170
Giving Your Horse
     Oral Medications...................171
How to Administer Eye
     Medications to Your Pet..........172
If Your Pet Gets into Poison...........173

Index 175

Acetaminophen

Tylenol®, paracetamol and APAP are other names for this medication.

How Is This Medication Useful?

- Acetaminophen is a pain reliever and fever reducer. It is important to know that dogs and cats have a higher normal body temperature (101°F-103°F) than humans. These temperatures are not considered to be fever in dogs and cats and should not be treated with anti-fever medications.
- Acetaminophen is not frequently used in animal patients, but may be useful when other pain relievers cause harm to the stomach and kidneys. Acetaminophen is not usually used alone in dogs, but is combined with a strong pain reliever called codeine.

Are There Conditions or Times When Its Use Might Cause More Harm Than Good?

- Acetaminophen should **NEVER be used in cats** as death may result.
- Acetaminophen is a human medication that should be used very carefully in treating dogs and should not be used at all in cats. Very small doses of acetaminophen (1/2 of a regular strength Tylenol®) can kill an adult cat.
- Acetaminophen should be used very carefully in animals with liver problems.
- Acetaminophen is used safely in pregnant humans, but should probably be used only with caution in pregnant animals.
- Acetaminophen should not be used with other pain relievers or fever reducers unless instructed by your veterinarian.
- If your animal has any of the above conditions, talk to your veterinarian about the potential risks of using the medication versus the benefits that it might have.

What Side Effects Can Be Seen With Its Use?

- Acetaminophen does not usually have side effects but some animals may experience stomach upset, kidney problems or blood cell problems.
- If too much acetaminophen is used, your pet could develop liver failure and severe blood problems.

How Should It Be Given?

- The successful outcome of your animal's treatment with this medication depends upon your commitment and ability to administer it exactly as the veterinarian has prescribed. Please do not skip doses or stop giving the medication. If you have difficulty giving doses consult your veterinarian or pharmacist who can offer administration techniques or change the dosage form to a type of medication that may be more acceptable to you and your animal.
- Some other drugs can interact with this medication so tell your veterinarian about any drugs or foods that you currently give your animal. Do not give new foods or medications without first asking your veterinarian.
- **Dogs**: Give this medication exactly as instructed by your veterinarian and do not miss any doses. If you see signs of blood in the stools or urine, or if you see vomiting, call your veterinarian immediately.
- Do not give this medication to cats as it will likely kill them.
- Keep this medication away from all children as overdoses can be poisonous.

What Other Information Is Important About This Medication?

- Capsules or tablets should be stored at room temperature.
- You should watch your pet for any signs of the side effects listed previously.
- There are many different brands and strengths of this medication. Do not buy an over the counter substitute without the advice of your veterinarian or pharmacist.

Acetazolamide

Diamox® is another name for this medication.

How Is This Medication Useful?

- Acetazolamide is primarily used to treat HYPP (hyperkalemic periodic paralysis) in Quarterhorses descended from the original horse ("Impressive") that had this disease.
- Acetazolamide may sometimes be used to treat glaucoma in animals.

Are There Conditions or Times When Its Use Might Cause More Harm Than Good?

- Acetazolamide should not be used in patients with liver or kidney disease, low blood sodium, low blood potassium or Addison's disease.
- Acetazolamide should not be used in patients who have lung problems or difficulty breathing as too much acid may build up in the lungs and blood.
- Acetazolamide should not be used in patients that are allergic to it or to drugs like it.
- Acetazolamide should be used with extreme caution in patients whose blood is too acidic (acidosis).
- Acetazolamide should be used with caution in diabetics as it may make blood sugar very high.
- Aspirin has a very low margin of safety in dogs and cats. The use of acetazolamide and aspirin together is not recommended in dogs or cats as this combination may make aspirin even less safe to use.
- Uric acid secretion is reduced with acetazolamide and may cause gout or certain kinds of kidney stones.
- This drug should be used cautiously in patients or by caregivers with known hypersensitivity to sulfas, as it is related to the sulfa drugs.
- Acetazolamide has caused birth defects and should not be used in pregnant or nursing animals.
- If your animal has any of the above conditions, talk to your veterinarian about the potential risks of using the medication versus the benefits that it might have.

What Side Effects Can Be Seen With Its Use?

- The primary adverse effect of acetazolamide in animals is stomach upset. This effect may be reduced by giving the medication with food.
- Other side effects reported include sleepiness, confusion, staggering, and seizures.
- Anemias have been reported after chronic administration of acetazolamide.
- Patients with hypercalciuria (too much calcium in the urine) are more likely to have kidney stone formation from acetazolamide.
- Low potassium may result and the risk is increased in the presence of potassium wasting drugs like diuretics such as furosemide (Lasix®).
- High blood sugar can sometimes result from the low potassium.
- If you notice any signs of panting, weakness, disorientation or behavior changes you should notify your veterinarian immediately.

How Should It Be Given?

- Acetazolamide is usually given orally as a tablet or an oral liquid or paste.
- The successful outcome of your animal's treatment with this medication depends upon your commitment and ability to administer it exactly as the veterinarian has prescribed. Please do not skip doses or stop giving the medication. If you have difficulty giving doses consult your veterinarian or pharmacist who can offer administration techniques or change the dosage form to a type of medication that may be more acceptable to you and your animal.
- If you miss a dose of this medication you should give it as soon as you remember it, but if it is within a few hours of the regularly scheduled dose, wait and give it at the regular time. Do not double a dose as this can be toxic to your pet.
- Some other drugs can interact with this medication so tell your veterinarian about any drugs or foods that you currently give your animal. Do not give new foods or medications without first asking your veterinarian.
- **Dogs and Cats**: Dogs and cats may receive this drug for glaucoma orally three times daily.
- **Horses**: Horses receive this drug orally twice daily for prevention of HYPP episodes and may receive a higher dose during an HYPP crisis.

(Continued on following page)

VETERINARY DRUG HANDBOOK-Client Information Edition
Permission to photocopy for individual clients granted by Gigi Davidson and Donald C. Plumb © 2003

Acetazolamide

(continued)

What Other Information Is Important About This Medication?

- Acetazolamide should be stored at room temperature in a tight, light resistant, childproof container away from all children and other household pets.
- This medication is being given to control your horse's paralysis episodes. Give it as instructed by your veterinarian and do not miss any doses especially during trailering or other times of immobility.
- You should provide your horse with a regular feeding and exercise and avoid water deprivation or fasting. Your horse is likely to have a relapse if confined for a long period (>2hrs) in a stall or a trailer. You should feed low potassium containing foods such as alfalfa mixed with grass or oat hay and grains, especially oats. You should avoid rapid changes in your horse's diet.
- You should remove any salt licks and mineral supplements from your horse's paddock and consult your veterinarian prior to administering any new feeds or mineral supplements.
- This medication may be difficult to obtain in the large quantities (16-20 tablets daily) needed by adult horses. Contact your pharmacist well ahead of time (at least one week) in order to obtain refills without missing doses.

Albuterol

Proventil® and Torpex® are other names for this medication

How Is This Medication Useful?

- Albuterol is a drug which acts to relax the muscles of the airways and is used to improve breathing. It is used in animals for relief of cough caused by asthma and other conditions.

Are There Conditions or Times When Its Use Might Cause More Harm Than Good?

- Albuterol can sometimes over-stimulate the brain and the heart. It should not be used in animals with heart disease, high blood pressure, seizures, thyroid conditions or diabetes. Albuterol has also caused low blood sugar and fast heartbeat in the fetuses of mothers taking the medication. It should not be used in a pregnant animal unless you and your veterinarian decide that the benefit to the mother is worth more than the risk to the babies.
- If your animal has any of the above conditions, talk to your veterinarian about the potential risks of using the medication versus the benefits that it might have.

What Side Effects Can Be Seen With Its Use?

- The most common side effects seen with albuterol are nervousness, shaking, fast heartbeat, and dizziness.
- In horses, the most common side effects are sweating, muscle tremors and mild excitement. All of these side effects usually go away within 30 minutes of giving the dose. If they do not, you should call your veterinarian.

How Should It Be Given?

- The Torpex® inhaler should be shaken 2-3 times before using. Give the inhaler a test puff away from the horse's face. Be careful to avoid inhaling the mist yourself. Insert the tip into the nostril and deliver 3 puffs. If the medication does not work in a few minutes, you may give 3 more puffs. Do not give more than 24 puffs in a day and not more than 5 days in a row.
- The successful outcome of your animal's treatment with this medication depends upon your commitment and ability to administer it exactly as the veterinarian has prescribed. Please do not skip doses or stop giving the medication. If you have difficulty giving doses consult your veterinarian or pharmacist who can offer administration techniques or change the dosage form to a type of medication that may be more acceptable to you and your animal.

- Some other drugs can interact with this medication so tell your veterinarian about any drugs or foods that you currently give your animal. Do not give new foods or medications without first asking your veterinarian.
- **Dogs and Cats:** Give this drug exactly as instructed by your veterinarian. It will help your pet breathe better. If you miss a dose, do not double it the next time as it will probably cause the side effects mentioned above. It may be given as an oral liquid, a tablet, as an aerosol or in a special machine (nebulizer) with a special mask which will allow your pet to breathe the medication directly into its lungs. It is usually given up to four times in one day. If you notice any deterioration in your pet's breathing or changes in behavior, call your veterinarian immediately.
- **Horses:** Horses usually receive albuterol as an inhaler (Torpex®). It is given as an aerosol into the lungs through a special inhaler. Horses receive 3 puffs per dose up to 4 treatments daily for no more than 5 days in a row.

What Other Information Is Important About This Medication?

- This medication should be stored at room temperature and in the original packaging provided by your veterinarian until immediately before use. You should watch your pet for all the above side effects mentioned above.
- **Dogs and Cats:** You should not discontinue the use of this drug without the advice of your veterinarian.
- **Horses**: This drug is a Class 3 drug in the ARCI (Animal Racing Commissioners International) uniform classification guidelines. It is banned by the ASHA as a prohibited substance in performance horses. You should keep it away from your horse's eyes when administering. You should also avoid inhaling the mist yourself.

VETERINARY DRUG HANDBOOK-Client Information Edition
Permission to photocopy for individual clients granted by Gigi Davidson and Donald C. Plumb © 2003

Allopurinol

Zyloprim® is another name for this medication.

How Is This Medication Useful?

- Allopurinol is useful in preventing the buildup of a substance called uric acid that causes gout and certain types of kidney stones.

Are There Conditions or Times When Its Use Might Cause More Harm Than Good?

- Allopurinol is removed from the body by the liver and the kidneys. This drug should be used with extreme caution in animals with kidney or liver disease. If your animal has any of the above conditions, talk to your veterinarian about the potential risks of using the medication versus the benefits that it might have.

What Side Effects Can Be Seen With Its Use?

- While alloupurinol can cause blood problems and liver problems in people, these effects are not seen very often in animals.
- While normal doses of allopurinol are used to prevent a certain kind of kidney stone (urate) high doses of allopurinol can cause formation of a different kind of kidney stone (xanthine).
- Some animals are allergic to allopurinol and the drug should not be used in these animals.

How Should It Be Given?

- The successful outcome of your animal's treatment with this medication depends upon your commitment and ability to administer it exactly as the veterinarian has prescribed. Please do not skip doses or stop giving the medication. If you have difficulty giving doses consult your veterinarian or pharmacist who can offer administration techniques or change the dosage form to a type of medication that may be more acceptable to you and your animal.
- Some other drugs can interact with this medication so tell your veterinarian about any drugs or foods that you currently give your animal. Do not give new foods or medications without first asking your veterinarian.

- **Birds**: This medication is usually given over three doses in a day or it may be added to your bird's drinking water. You should make fresh solutions daily if you are giving the medicine in the water. You should watch your pet for any signs of rash or unusual tiredness and report them to your veterinarian immediately.
- **Dogs and Cats:** This medication is usually given to dogs and cats over two to three doses in a day. You should give it after meals unless your veterinarian has told you otherwise. Your veterinarian may give other medications to increase the effectiveness of this one. Please give all medication exactly as your veterinarian has prescribed and do not miss any doses. You should watch your pet for any signs of rash or unusual tiredness and report them to your veterinarian immediately.

What Other Information Is Important About This Medication?

- This medication should be stored at room temperature in a well-closed container. This as all medications should be kept out of the reach of children and pets.

Altrenogest

Regumate® is another name for this medication.

How Is This Medication Useful?

- Altrenogest is a hormone that is given to horses to keep them from cycling or if they are already pregnant, to keep them from losing the foal.

Are There Conditions or Times When Its Use Might Cause More Harm Than Good?

- Altrenogest should not be used in horses that are intended for human food.
- Although it is rarely used in dogs, it may be used to increase the fertility of female dogs. It may cause a condition called pyometra (infected uterus). If your dog has a fever (103°-104°F) while on altrenogest, you should contact your veterinarian immediately.
- Altrenogest should not be used in animals with an infected uterus.
- Altrenogest can also disrupt the hormonal cycles of human females. It may stop the effectiveness of birth control pills. If you are a female, you should wear nitrile gloves while handling this medication. If you spill it on yourself, you should call your gynecologist.
- The manufacturer of altrenogest recommends that certain persons not handle this product:
  o Women who are pregnant or may be pregnant
  o Anyone with blood clots or a history of blood clot
  o Anyone with hardening of the arteries or a history of stroke
  o Women with breast cancer or a history of breast cancer
  o Women with estrogen dependent cancerous tumors
  o Women with undiagnosed vaginal bleeding
  o Women who had tumors that developed while taking estrogens or oral contraceptives.
- If you or your animal has any of the above conditions, talk to your veterinarian about the potential risks of using the medication versus the benefits that it might have.

What Side Effects Can Be Seen With Its Use?

- When used appropriately there are usually few side effects seen in horses.
- Changes in blood calcium or potassium are possible.
- Increases in enzymes (AST and alkaline phosphatase) that can be released when liver damage occurs have been seen.

- Mares who have chronic uterine infections may have those infections get worse if treated with altrenogest.

How Should It Be Given?

- The successful outcome of your animal's treatment with this medication depends upon your commitment and ability to administer it exactly as the veterinarian has prescribed. Please do not skip doses or stop giving the medication. If you have difficulty giving doses consult your veterinarian or pharmacist who can offer administration techniques or change the dosage form to a type of medication that may be more acceptable to you and your animal.
- If you miss a dose of this medication you should give it as soon as you remember it, but if it is within a few hours of the regularly scheduled dose, wait and give it at the regular time. Do not double a dose as this can be toxic to your pet.
- Some other drugs can interact with this medication so tell your veterinarian about any drugs or foods that you currently give your animal. Do not give new foods or medications without first asking your veterinarian.
- **Dogs and Cats**: Altrenogest is rarely given to dogs, but may be used in female dogs that have fertility problems.
- **Horses**: Horses usually receive altrenogest orally once daily mixed in the feed.

What Other Information Is Important About This Medication?

- Altrenogest should be stored in a tight, light resistant, childproof container away from all children and other household pets.
- It is not supplied in a child-resistant bottle and frequently drips down the side when removing a dose. You should always wear gloves when handling this medication. As this is a very oily drug, lots of detergent and water may be required for clean up.

Aminocaproic Acid

Amicar® is another name for this medication.

How Is This Medication Useful?

- Aminocaproic acid is used to help treat nerve degeneration in dogs. It helps stop the inflammation process that damages nerves. It may also be used if your pet has a blood clot in the eye.

Are There Conditions or Times When Its Use Might Cause More Harm Than Good?

- Even though this drug is sometimes used to treat blood clots in the eye, it can also cause blood clots in parts of the body where they are dangerous.
- If your pet has liver, heart or kidney disease, this drug should be used with extreme caution.
- Some research has shown that this drug will cause birth defects. It should probably not be used in pregnancy. It also can get into the mother's milk and should not be given to mothers who are still nursing babies.
- If your animal has any of the above conditions, talk to your veterinarian about the potential risks of using the medication versus the benefits that it might have.

What Side Effects Can Be Seen With Its Use?

- The most common side effect seen in dogs is stomach upset.
- This drug may also cause the formation of blood clots in your pet's blood vessels.
- This drug may cause the level of potassium in the blood to become too high in animals with kidney disease.
- If the dose is too high, aminocaproic acid may cause your pet to have seizures.

How Should It Be Given?

- The successful outcome of your animal's treatment with this medication depends upon your commitment and ability to administer it exactly as the veterinarian has prescribed. Please do not skip doses or stop giving the medication. If you have difficulty giving doses consult your veterinarian or pharmacist who can offer administration techniques or change the dosage form to a type of medication that may be more acceptable to you and your animal.

- Some other drugs can interact with this medication so tell your veterinarian about any drugs or foods that you currently give your animal. Do not give new foods or medications without first asking your veterinarian.
- **Dogs**: This medication is usually mixed into an oral liquid for dogs and is flavored with a multivitamin to improve the taste. Most dogs will start to get better within 8 weeks of staring this medicine. You should watch your dog for any signs of stomach upset, seizures or any abnormal bleeding. If you see any of these symptoms, you should tell your veterinarian immediately.

What Other Information Is Important About This Medication?

- This drug is very expensive, but should significantly help your dog's nervous system degeneration. Do not try to skip doses or lower the dose to save money as this will only cause your dog's condition to worsen and the medication will have to be given even longer.
- This drug should be stored at room temperature and protected from extreme heat or freezing.

Aminophylline

Slo-phylline® is another name for this medication.

How Is This Medication Useful?

- This medication is used to relax airways and help animals breathe better. It is used in conditions such as asthma or heaves. It is sometimes used with other medications in the treatment of heart failure.

Are There Conditions or Times When Its Use Might Cause More Harm Than Good?

- Aminophylline can cause the heart to beat too fast. It should be used with extreme caution in animals with irregular heartbeats or heart disease.
- Aminophylline might also worsen the conditions of stomach ulcers, thyroid disease, kidney or liver disease or high blood pressure.
- If your animal has any of the above conditions, talk to your veterinarian about the potential risks of using the medication versus the benefits that it might have.
- Aminophylline might take longer to get out of the bodies of very young or very old animals and should be used carefully in these patients.

What Side Effects Can Be Seen With Its Use?

- The most common side effects from aminophylline are stomach upset and fast heartbeat. At the beginning of treatment, your animal may experience nervousness and stomach upset but these side effects usually go away as your animal's body gets used to the medication.
- Aminophylline may cause some animals to eat more, drink more and urinate more.
- Horses may become more nervous, have a fast heartbeat, sweat and be unstable on their feet.
- In higher doses, some animals may have seizures.
- If you see any of these side effects in your animal, you should tell your veterinarian immediately.

How Should It Be Given?

- Aminophylline should be given exactly as your veterinarian has told you. It can be dangerous in doses that are too high. You should never skip doses. If you accidentally forget to give a dose, you should never double the next dose to make up for it. The successful outcome of your animal's treatment with this medication depends upon your commitment and ability to administer it exactly as the veterinarian has prescribed. If you have difficulty giving any doses, please do not skip doses or stop giving the medication. Consult your veterinarian or pharmacist who can offer administration techniques or change the dosage form to a type of medication that may be more acceptable to you and your animal.
- Some other drugs can interact with this medication so tell your veterinarian about any drugs or foods that you currently give your animal. Do not give new foods or medications without first asking your veterinarian.
- **Dogs and Cats**: Aminophylline is usually given to dogs and cats twice or three times daily. It should be given exactly as the veterinarian has instructed. It is not unusual at the beginning of treatment for animals to experience nervousness or upset stomach from this drug. These side effects should go away in a short time. If these effects return after a while, you should tell your veterinarian immediately.
- **Horses**: This drug is banned for use in horses that are going to show or race. It is usually given two or three times daily and may be mixed in the feed. Horses may initially show nervousness, sweating, fast heartbeat and may be unstable on their feet. These side effects will usually go away with time.

What Other Information Is Important About This Medication?

- This medication should be stored at room temperature and protected from extreme heat or freezing.
- **Horses**: This drug is banned by the ASHA and should not be used in show or race horses while they are performing.

VETERINARY DRUG HANDBOOK-Client Information Edition
Permission to photocopy for individual clients granted by Gigi Davidson and Donald C. Plumb © 2003

Amitriptyline

Elavil® is another name for this medication.

How Is This Medication Useful?

- This medication is used to make your pet feel less anxious when it is away from you (separation anxiety) or during certain frightening circumstances (thunderstorms, fireworks).
- Amitriptyline is also useful in stopping some bad behaviors such as urine spraying or excessive biting and chewing of skin.
- It is also used in birds to stop behavior problems such as feather picking.

Are There Conditions or Times When Its Use Might Cause More Harm Than Good?

- Amitriptyline may cause dangerous side effects if mixed with certain chemicals such as those found in tick collars.
- Certain foods such as aged cheese may also cause this drug to have bad side effects.
- This medication should not be used in pregnant animals as it has caused birth defects.
- Amitriptyline crosses into mother's milk and should not be given to mothers who are still nursing babies.
- This medication should be used with caution in diabetic animals as it may alter usual insulin requirements. If this medication is suddenly stopped after being given regularly for a long time, your pet may experience vomiting, anxiety and shaking.
- If your animal has any of the above conditions, talk to your veterinarian about the potential risks of using the medication versus the benefits that it might have.

What Side Effects Can Be Seen With Its Use?

- The most common side effects from amitriptyline are drowsiness, constipation, and dry mouth. Amitriptyline may also cause blood sugar to either increase or decrease in diabetic patients.
- Very high doses of amitriptyline can cause severe damage to the heart.

How Should It Be Given?

- The successful outcome of your animal's treatment with this medication depends upon your commitment and ability to administer it exactly as the veterinarian has prescribed. Please do not skip doses or stop giving the medication. If you have difficulty giving doses consult your veterinarian or pharmacist who can offer administration techniques or change the dosage form to a type of medication that may be more acceptable to you and your animal.
- Some other drugs can interact with this medication so tell your veterinarian about any drugs or foods that you currently give your animal. Do not give new foods or medications without first asking your veterinarian.
- **Dogs and Cats:** This medication is usually given to dogs and cats one to two times daily. It may take several weeks before changes in behavior are seen. Do not skip doses. If a dose is missed, do not double doses to catch up as this may increase the undesirable side effects. When the desired effect is reached with this drug, it must not be stopped suddenly. The drug must be tapered off slowly or the animal may suffer uncomfortable symptoms of withdrawal.
- **Birds**: Amitriptyline must be mixed into a special dosage form when used in birds because the tablets are too strong for birds. Most birds will receive a liquid form that should be stored exactly as the pharmacist has recommended.
- **Horses:** This drug is banned by AHSA and should not be used in horses that are going to race or be shown.

What Other Information Is Important About This Medication?

- Tablets and capsules of this medication should be stored at room temperature. Liquids should be stored exactly as the pharmacist has recommended and discarded by the date shown on the prescription bottle.
- Overdoses of amitriptyline can be very serious in both humans and animals, be very careful to keep out of the reach of children and animals.

Amlodipine

Norvasc® is another name for this medication.

How Is This Medication Useful?

- This medication works on the heart and blood vessels to help lower blood pressure. High blood pressure in animals can cause kidney damage and blindness. High blood pressure usually occurs more in cats than in dogs.

Are There Conditions or Times When Its Use Might Cause More Harm Than Good?

- Amlodipine has strong effects on the heart and should be used carefully in animals with heart failure.
- Amlodipine is also removed from the body by the liver, and should be used carefully in animals with liver disease.
- This drug has also caused birth defects and should not be used in pregnant or nursing animals.
- It should be used carefully in combination with other drugs that lower blood pressure to prevent the blood pressure from becoming too low.
- If your animal has any of the above conditions, talk to your veterinarian about the potential risks of using the medication versus the benefits that it might have.

What Side Effects Can Be Seen With Its Use?

- Amlodipine does not have many side effects in animals. Headache is a common side effect when used in humans.
- This drug can also cause the blood to take longer to clot when used in dogs. For this reason, it should be used very carefully in combination with other drugs that thin the blood such as warfarin or aspirin.

How Should It Be Given?

- The successful outcome of your animal's treatment with this medication depends upon your commitment and ability to administer it exactly as the veterinarian has prescribed. Please do not skip doses or stop giving the medication. If you have difficulty giving doses consult your veterinarian or pharmacist who can offer administration techniques or change the dosage form to a type of medication that may be more acceptable to you and your animal.
- Some other drugs can interact with this medication so tell your veterinarian about any drugs or foods that you currently give your animal. Do not give new foods or medications without first asking your veterinarian.
- **Dogs and Cats:** Amlodipine is usually given by mouth to cats and dogs once daily. It can be given with food. You will need to take your pet back to the veterinarian for blood pressure checks and eye exams to make sure that the medication is working.

What Other Information Is Important About This Medication?

- This medication is available as a diamond shaped tablet. Because of this shape, the tablet may be hard to split into halves or quarters. Because cats can be very sensitive to this drug, it is best to have your pharmacist make you special capsules that contain exactly the right dose.
- Try not to skip doses. If you miss a dose, give it as soon as you remember it, but never double a dose to make up for missed ones as this may increase the side effects.

Ammonium Chloride

Uroeze® is another name for this medication.

How Is This Medication Useful?

- This medication is used to prevent the formation of certain kinds of kidney and bladder stones. Ammonium chloride makes the urine more acidic and prevents formation of these stones.
- Ammonium chloride can also be used to increase the elimination of certain kinds of toxins or drugs from the body through the urine.
- It may also be used in combination with certain antibiotic medications to increase the effect of the antibiotic against certain bacteria in the urine.

Are There Conditions or Times When Its Use Might Cause More Harm Than Good?

- Because the liver must be functioning well to eliminate ammonia-containing substances, this drug should be used with extreme caution if you pet has liver problems.
- Because ammonium chloride can cause an increase in acidity in the whole body, not just the urine, it should be used very carefully in patients that have lung problems. The lungs are used to breathe off carbon dioxide, another acidic substance that can accumulate in the body.
- If your animal has any of the above conditions, talk to your veterinarian about the potential risks of using the medication versus the benefits that it might have.

What Side Effects Can Be Seen With Its Use?

- When given by mouth, ammonium chloride can sometimes cause stomach upset and vomiting. Giving the medication with food will sometimes decrease this side effect.
- Injectable forms of ammonium chloride are very irritating and cause pain and stinging at the injection site.
- Very high doses of ammonium chloride can be dangerous. If your animal seems to be panting excessively, breathing too fast or seems unusually drowsy, you should contact your veterinarian immediately.

How Should It Be Given?

- The successful outcome of your animal's treatment with this medication depends upon your commitment and ability to administer it exactly as the veterinarian has prescribed. Please do not skip doses or stop giving the medication. If you have difficulty giving doses consult your veterinarian or pharmacist who can offer administration techniques or change the dosage form to a type of medication that may be more acceptable to you and your animal.
- Some other drugs can interact with this medication so tell your veterinarian about any drugs or foods that you currently give your animal. Do not give new foods or medications without first asking your veterinarian.
- **Dogs and Cats**: Dogs usually receive ammonium chloride orally in three to four daily doses and cats usually receive the drug twice daily.
- **Horses**: Horses usually receive ammonium chloride as a powder to be sprinkled over the feed once daily.

What Other Information Is Important About This Medication?

- This medication should be stored at room temperature and protected from extreme heat and freezing. This drug should be kept away from fertilizers and other strong oxidizing substances (*e.g.*, potassium chlorate) as the combination can be highly explosive.
- **Dogs and Cats:** Your veterinarian will ask you to monitor the acidity of your pet's urine to make sure the drug is working. You can purchase pH tape from your veterinarian or pharmacy and check the urine periodically to make sure that the pH is less than 6.5.
- **Horses**: Ammonium chloride may mask the presence of banned drugs used in performance horses so use of ammonium chloride is prohibited in any racing or showing animals.

Amoxicillin

Amoxil®, Amoxitabs®, Trimox® and Wymox® are other names for this medication.

How Is This Medication Useful?

- Amoxicillin is a broad spectrum penicillin-class antibiotic used to treat infections in dogs and cats.

Are There Conditions or Times When Its Use Might Cause More Harm Than Good?

- Amoxicillin is a very safe antibiotic but may cause serious problems in animals with penicillin allergies.
- Horses may develop severe diarrhea with subsequent colic when amoxicillin is given orally; use with caution.
- Rabbits may also develop severe diarrhea when given amoxicillin orally. You should never give antibiotics orally to your rabbit unless a veterinarian has specifically directed you to do so.
- If your animal has allergies to penicillins or has had bad reactions to penicillins in the past, talk to your veterinarian about the potential risks of using the medication versus the benefits that it might have for your animal.
- You should always give all of the medication as directed by your veterinarian. If the entire course of treatment is not finished, the germ causing the infection may become stronger than the antibiotics and cause a worsening infection.

What Side Effects Can Be Seen With Its Use?

- Most animals (not horses or rabbits) tolerate amoxicillin very well, but it may cause decreased appetite, vomiting and diarrhea. Giving this medication with food may decrease the occurrences of reduced appetite and vomiting.

How Should It Be Given?

- The successful outcome of your animal's treatment with this medication depends upon your commitment and ability to administer it exactly as the veterinarian has prescribed. Please do not skip doses or stop giving the medication. If you have difficulty giving doses consult your veterinarian or pharmacist who can offer administration techniques or change the dosage form to a type of medication that may be more acceptable to you and your animal.

- If you miss a dose of this medication you should give it as soon as you remember it, but if it is within a few hours of the regularly scheduled dose, wait and give it at the regular time. Do not double a dose as this can be toxic to your pet.
- Some other drugs can interact with this medication so tell your veterinarian about any drugs or foods that you currently give your animal. Do not give new foods or medications without first asking your veterinarian.
- **Dogs and Cats:** This medication is usually given orally twice daily to dogs and cats as an oral tablet or liquid. In the veterinary hospital it may be given as an injection under the skin twice daily.
- **Ferrets**: This medication has been given to ferrets orally two to three times daily for infection.
- **Birds**: This medication has been given to birds orally three to four times daily for infection.
- **Horses**: This drug has been given orally to horses for severe respiratory infections, but may cause severe diarrhea and subsequent colic or death.

What Other Information Is Important About This Medication?

- Amoxicillin should be stored in a tight, light resistant, childproof container away from all children and other household pets.
- Oral liquids should be shaken well, stored in the refrigerator, and not used after 14 days.

VETERINARY DRUG HANDBOOK-Client Information Edition
Permission to photocopy for individual clients granted by Gigi Davidson and Donald C. Plumb © 2003

Amoxicillin/Clavulanate

Clavamox® and Augmentin® are other names for this medication.

How Is This Medication Useful?

- Amoxicillin/Clavulanate is a broad spectrum antibiotic used to treat infections in dogs and cats. Amoxicillin is a type of penicillin that is often used alone. Clavulanate is added to increase its effectiveness against certain types of bacteria.

Are There Conditions or Times When Its Use Might Cause More Harm Than Good?

- Amoxicillin/Clavulanate is a very safe antibiotic but may cause serious problems in animals with penicillin allergies. If your animal has allergies to penicillins or has had bad reactions to penicillins in the past, talk to your veterinarian about the potential risks of using the medication versus the benefits that it might have for your animal.
- Amoxicillin/Clavulanate has caused rare liver problems in humans and this effect has been reported in a few dogs. Please let your veterinarian know if your pet has or has had severe liver problems.
- Horses may develop severe diarrhea with subsequent colic when amoxicillin/clavulanate is given orally; use is not recommended in this species.
- Rabbits can also develop severe diarrhea after given oral amoxicillin/clavulanate. You should not give your rabbit oral antibiotics without your veterinarian's advice.
- You should always give all of the medication as directed by your veterinarian. If the entire course of treatment is not finished, the germ causing the infection may become stronger than the antibiotics and cause a worsening infection.

What Side Effects Can Be Seen With Its Use?

- Most animals (not horses) tolerate amoxicillin/clavulanate very well, but it may cause decreased appetite, vomiting and diarrhea. Giving this medication with food may decrease the occurrences of reduced appetite and vomiting.
- Very high doses of this drug may cause your dog to become dizzy. If you notice any behavior change or dizziness in your pet, you should contact your veterinarian immediately.

How Should It Be Given?

- The successful outcome of your animal's treatment with this medication depends upon your commitment and ability to administer it exactly as the veterinarian has prescribed. Please do not skip doses or stop giving the medication. If you have difficulty giving doses consult your veterinarian or pharmacist who can offer administration techniques or change the dosage form to a type of medication that may be more acceptable to you and your animal.
- If you miss a dose of this medication you should give it as soon as you remember it, but if it is within a few hours of the regularly scheduled dose, wait and give it at the regular time. Do not double a dose as this can be toxic to your pet.
- Some other drugs can interact with this medication so tell your veterinarian about any drugs or foods that you currently give your animal. Do not give new foods or medications without first asking your veterinarian.
- **Dogs and Cats:** This medication is usually given orally twice daily to dogs and cats as an oral tablet or liquid.
- **Ferrets**: This medication has been given to ferrets orally two to three times daily for infection.
- **Birds**: This medication has been given to birds orally three to four times daily for infection.
- **Horses**: This drug has been given to foals in an injectable form. This drug should not be given orally to horses as it may cause a severe diarrhea and subsequent colic or death.

What Other Information Is Important About This Medication?

- Amoxicillin/Clavulanate should be stored in a tight, light resistant, child proof container away from all children and other household pets.
- Tablets should not be split prior to use as air will cause them to rapidly deteriorate.
- Oral liquids should be shaken well, stored in the refrigerator, and not used after 10 days. They should be discarded if they turn yellow or brown.
- The human forms of this drug (Augmentin®) contain different amounts of clavulanate than the veterinary products. You should not use the human products in your pet without specific instructions from your veterinarian.

Ascorbic Acid

Vitamin C is another name for this medication.

How Is This Medication Useful?

- Vitamin C is necessary for all animals in order to maintain good nutrition and immune system function.
- Ascorbic acid is given to guinea pigs and some other animals as a dietary supplement to prevent scurvy. Like humans, Guinea pigs need vitamin C as they cannot create it like most other species.
- Sometimes ascorbic acid may be used to make the urine more acid to prevent stone formation or to increase the elimination of toxic drugs.
- Vitamin C injection is also a valuable antidote for horses that have been poisoned by eating Red Maple leaves.

Are There Conditions or Times When Its Use Might Cause More Harm Than Good?

- Large doses of vitamin C can mask the presence of sugar in the urine and may be dangerous for diabetics who use urine glucose tests to monitor their disease.
- Vitamin C may also inactivate the test that is used to check for blood in the stool.
- Animals with Copper Storage Disease (primarily Bedlington Terriers) should not receive vitamin C as it can worsen the condition.
- Because ascorbic acid makes the urine more acid, it can cause changes in the way a drug is eliminated from the body. Please tell your veterinarian about any other medications that your pet is receiving prior to using ascorbic acid.
- If your animal has any of the above conditions, talk to your veterinarian about the potential risks of using the medication versus the benefits that it might have.

What Side Effects Can Be Seen With Its Use?

- There are very few side effects from ascorbic acid but large doses can cause diarrhea.
- Very large doses of ascorbic acid can cause stone formation in the urine.

How Should It Be Given?

- The successful outcome of your animal's treatment with this medication depends upon your commitment and ability to administer it exactly as the veterinarian has prescribed. Please do not skip doses or stop giving the medication. If you have difficulty giving doses consult your veterinarian or pharmacist who can offer administration techniques or change the dosage form to a type of medication that may be more acceptable to you and your animal.
- If you miss a dose of this medication you should give it as soon as you remember it, but if it is within a few hours of the regularly scheduled dose, wait and give it at the regular time. Do not double a dose, as this can be toxic to your pet.
- Some other drugs can interact with this medication so tell your veterinarian about any drugs or foods that you currently give your animal. Do not give new foods or medications without first asking your veterinarian.
- **Dogs and Cats**: Dogs and cats usually receive this drug orally as a tablet twice daily.
- **Guinea Pigs**: Guinea pigs usually receive 200mg of ascorbic acid daily in their water bottles.
- **Horses:** Horses suffering from Red Maple leaf poisoning will receive vitamin C injection intravenously. Vitamin C may mask drug test results and should not be used in performance horses.
- **Cattle:** Vitamin C injection has been given to calves with certain kinds of skin diseases.

What Other Information Is Important About This Medication?

- Ascorbic acid is very sensitive to air and light and should be stored in a tight, light resistant, childproof container away from all children and other household pets. This medication will darken upon exposure to light, but color changes do not affect potency.
- Ascorbic acid injection should not be stored or opened after its expiration date as it decomposes to a substance that will build pressure in the vial and may cause the vial to burst.

VETERINARY DRUG HANDBOOK-Client Information Edition
Permission to photocopy for individual clients granted by Gigi Davidson and Donald C. Plumb © 2003

Aspirin

How Is This Medication Useful?

- Aspirin is used to treat pain, fever and to thin the blood in virtually all species of animals. It is used most commonly in animals to thin the blood to prevent blood clots. It is not used very commonly for pain as there are many other drugs that are safer and more effective than aspirin to treat pain in animals.

Are There Conditions or Times When Its Use Might Cause More Harm Than Good?

- Aspirin should be used very carefully in cats, only under the guidance and supervision of a veterinarian. Cats do not have the enzymes necessary to break down aspirin and rid it from the body.
- Aspirin is detoxified in the liver and the kidney and should be used very carefully in animals with liver or kidney problems.
- Aspirin thins the blood and should not be used in animals for at least one week prior to surgery. It should also be used with caution in animals who have bleeding tendencies or are anemic.
- Aspirin can also worsen ulcers and should not be used in animals with a history of ulcers.
- It has been shown to delay birth and should not be given to animals in the last stages of pregnancy.
- If your animal has any of the above conditions, talk to your veterinarian about the potential risks of using the medication versus the benefits that it might have.

What Side Effects Can Be Seen With Its Use?

- Aspirin can reduce the flow of blood to the stomach and intestines and can result in stomach pain and ulcers. Early signs of this adverse effect are vomiting, diarrhea or reluctance to eat. Giving aspirin with food can decrease the severity of these effects. Signs that aspirin is causing blood loss are black stools or vomit that looks like coffee grounds.
- Aspirin can also cause increases in blood sugar and should be used carefully in diabetic animals.
- If your pet shows any of these signs, contact your veterinarian immediately.

How Should It Be Given?

- The successful outcome of your animal's treatment with this medication depends upon your commitment and ability to administer it exactly as the veterinarian has prescribed. Please do not skip doses or stop giving the medication. If you have difficulty giving doses consult your veterinarian or pharmacist who can offer administration techniques or change the dosage form to a type of medication that may be more acceptable to you and your animal.
- Some other drugs can interact with this medication so tell your veterinarian about any drugs or foods that you currently give your animal. Drugs that decrease the acidity of the urine can decrease the effects of aspirin and drugs that increase the acidity of the urine can cause aspirin to become toxic. Other painkillers, fever medications and blood thinners should not generally be used at the same time as aspirin. Buffered aspirin may bind some antibiotics and may prevent them from working. Enteric coated aspirin is not usually effective in dogs and cats. Do not give new foods or medications without first asking your veterinarian.
- **Dogs and Cats:** Dogs usually receive aspirin two to three times daily. Cats rarely receive aspirin because they have great difficulties breaking it down and eliminating it. When used in cats, aspirin is usually given in small doses only once every two or three days.
- **Horses:** Horses usually get aspirin twice daily at first and then once it has achieved the desired effect the dose can be dropped to once daily.

What Other Information Is Important About This Medication?

- Animals receiving this medication will need to be monitored carefully by their veterinarian to make sure there are no ill effects on the blood or intestinal tract.
- Aspirin should be stored in light-resistant, airtight containers. Once aspirin takes on a vinegar-like odor, it will no longer achieve the desired effects.
- **Dogs and Cats:** Aspirin should be used only under the guidance of a veterinarian in dogs and cats.
- **Horses:** The use of aspirin is prohibited in horses that are racing or showing during therapy.

Atenolol

Tenormin® is another name for this medication.

How Is This Medication Useful?

- Atenolol is used to treat heart disease in cats and dogs. Atenolol works by slowing the heart and making it work more efficiently. It has also been used to lower blood pressure in dogs and cats.

Are There Conditions or Times When Its Use Might Cause More Harm Than Good?

- Animals with heart block or very slow heart rates may have problems taking this drug.
- Atenolol may also have some effects on the lungs. If your pet has asthma or other lung disease, please talk to your veterinarian before using this drug.
- If your animal has any of the above conditions, talk to your veterinarian about the potential risks of using the medication versus the benefits that it might have.

What Side Effects Can Be Seen With Its Use?

- This drug may cause your pet to become very tired. It may also slow the heartbeat too much if the dose is too high for your pet.
- Some dogs experience diarrhea while on this drug.
- If your pet has been on atenolol for a long time, you should not stop giving the drug suddenly or your pet may experience worse problems.

How Should It Be Given?

- The successful outcome of your animal's treatment with this medication depends upon your commitment and ability to administer it exactly as the veterinarian has prescribed. Please do not skip doses or stop giving the medication. If you have difficulty giving doses consult your veterinarian or pharmacist who can offer administration techniques or change the dosage form to a type of medication that may be more acceptable to you and your animal.
- If you miss a dose of this medication you should give it as soon as you remember it, but if it is within a few hours of the regularly scheduled dose, wait and give it at the regular time. Do not double a dose as this can be toxic to your pet.

- Some other drugs can interact with this medication so tell your veterinarian about any drugs or foods that you currently give your animal. Do not give new foods or medications without first asking your veterinarian.
- **Dogs and Cats**: Atenolol is usually given orally once or twice daily to dogs and once daily to cats.
- **Horses**: Atenolol is not typically given to horses and is considered a Class 3 drug by the Association of Racing Commissioners International.
- **Ferrets**: Atenolol has been given orally to ferrets once daily for heart disease.

What Other Information Is Important About This Medication?

- Atenolol should be stored in a tight, light resistant, child proof container away from all children and other household pets. If your pharmacist has compounded a special formulation for you, please observe the noted expiration dates for the product.
- This medication will probably need to be given for the rest of your animal's life. Please take your pet back to the veterinarian as instructed for very important follow up visits.

VETERINARY DRUG HANDBOOK-Client Information Edition
Permission to photocopy for individual clients granted by Gigi Davidson and Donald C. Plumb © 2003

Azathioprine

Imuran® is another name for this medication.

How Is This Medication Useful?

- Azathioprine is used to treat diseases and disorders caused by an overactive immune system. Azathioprine works by supressing the immune system.

Are There Conditions or Times When Its Use Might Cause More Harm Than Good?

- Azathioprine is cleared from the body by the liver and is used very carefully in animals with liver problems.
- Azathioprine should not be used in pregnant animals as it may cause birth defects.
- Azathioprine stops the bone marrow from producing blood cells. Cats are very susceptible to this effect and azathioprine is generally not recommended for use in cats.
- Azathioprine may also increase the risk of cancer later on in life.
- If your animal has any of the above conditions, talk to your veterinarian about the potential risks of using the medication versus the benefits that it might have.

What Side Effects Can Be Seen With Its Use?

- Azathioprine suppresses the bone marrow from producing blood cells and can cause anemias.
- Azathioprine can also cause damage to the liver and pancreas, especially in dogs.
- Because azathioprine suppresses the immune system, your pet may be more susceptible to infections.
- Azathioprine should not be stopped suddenly in animals who have been taking it as their immune systems are likely to overreact and cause the disease or disorder to start again.
- Azathioprine can also slow down the immune system of the humans who are giving it to their pets, so you should always wear gloves and wash your hands afterwards when giving this drug.

How Should It Be Given?

- The successful outcome of your animal's treatment with this medication depends upon your commitment and ability to administer it exactly as the veterinarian has prescribed. Please do not skip doses or stop giving the medication. If you have difficulty giving doses consult your veterinarian or pharmacist who can offer administration techniques or change the dosage

form to a type of medication that may be more acceptable to you and your animal.
- Some other drugs can interact with this medication so tell your veterinarian about any drugs or foods that you currently give your animal. Do not give new foods or medications without first asking your veterinarian.
- Humans should wear gloves when giving this drug and wash their hands afterwards as this drug can suppress the immune system of anyone exposed to it.
- If you miss a dose of this medication you should give it as soon as you remember it, but if it is within a few hours of the regularly scheduled dose wait until the regular time. Do not double the dose of azathioprine as it can be very toxic if overdosed.
- **Dogs**: Give this drug exactly as instructed by your veterinarian. Dogs usually receive this medication once daily at first and then the dose is given every other day.
- **Cats**: Azathioprine can severely affect the production of blood cells in cats and is generally not used in this species. If your veterinarian does decide to use this drug in your cat, you should give it exactly as the veterinarian has recommended. You will need to watch your cat very closely for signs of infection or bleeding that might occur as a result of treatment with azathioprine.

What Other Information Is Important About This Medication?

- The effects of azathioprine on your pet's disease may take as long as 6 weeks to occur. Do not discontinue this medication without guidance from your veterinarian as suddenly stopping azathioprine may make your pet get worse.
- Your veterinarian will need to check your pet's blood every 1-2 weeks when first starting this medication. Do not miss these important followup visits with your veterinarian.
- Azathioprine should always be handled with gloves and kept away from children and other pets.
- Azathioprine should be protected from light and moisture.

Baclofen

Lioresal® is another name for this medication.

How Is This Medication Useful?

- Baclofen is a muscle relaxant that may be useful in dogs who have difficulty urinating.

Are There Conditions or Times When Its Use Might Cause More Harm Than Good?

- Baclofen should not be used in cats.
- This drug should generally not be used in dogs who have or have ever had a seizure.
- Baclofen causes drowsiness and is not recommended for use in working animals that need to remain alert.
- This medication has caused birth defects and should only be used in pregnancy after careful consultation with your veterinarian.
- If your animal has any of the above conditions, talk to your veterinarian about the potential risks of using the medication versus the benefits that it might have.

What Side Effects Can Be Seen With Its Use?

- Baclofen usually causes drowsiness in most dogs.
- Baclofen may also cause weakness, itching and stomach upset in your dog.
- When discontinuing the use of baclofen, the drug should be tapered off gradually as hallucinations and seizures may occur if the drug is stopped too suddenly.

How Should It Be Given?

- The successful outcome of your animal's treatment with this medication depends upon your commitment and ability to administer it exactly as the veterinarian has prescribed. Please do not skip doses or stop giving the medication. If you have difficulty giving doses consult your veterinarian or pharmacist who can offer administration techniques or change the dosage form to a type of medication that may be more acceptable to you and your animal.
- If you miss a dose of this medication you should give it as soon as you remember it, but if it is within a few hours of the regularly scheduled dose, wait and give it at the regular time. Do not double a dose as this can be toxic to your pet.

- Some other drugs can interact with this medication so tell your veterinarian about any drugs or foods that you currently give your animal. Do not give new foods or medications without first asking your veterinarian.
- Do not stop giving this drug suddenly or your dog may experience hallucinations and seizures.
- **Dogs**: Baclofen is usually given orally as a tablet or a specially formulated liquid three times daily.
- **Cats**: Baclofen should not be given to cats.
- **Horses**: Baclofen has been given orally to horses and is considered a Class 4 drug by the Association of Racing Commissioners International.

What Other Information Is Important About This Medication?

- Baclofen should be stored in a tight, light resistant, childproof container away from all children and other household pets.

Benazepril

Lotensin® is another name for this medication.

How Is This Medication Useful?

- Benazepril is used to treat heart failure, high blood pressure and some forms of kidney disease in dogs and cats.

Are There Conditions or Times When Its Use Might Cause More Harm Than Good?

- Benazepril must be converted to the active drug, benazeprilat, by the liver. If your pet has severe liver disease, this drug may not work effectively.
- Benazepril should be used with caution in patients with very low sodium.
- This drug should not be used in patients with lupus.
- Benazepril has caused problems in pregnant humans and lab animals and should probably not be used in pregnancy.
- Benazepril does not cross into milk and can probably be used safely in nursing mothers.
- Benazepril can cause an increase in blood potassium levels if used with potassium or potassium sparing diuretics (spironolactone).
- If your animal has any of the above conditions, talk to your veterinarian about the potential risks of using the medication versus the benefits that it might have.

What Side Effects Can Be Seen With Its Use?

- Benazepril has few side effects but the most commonly reported ones are lack of appetite, vomiting and diarrhea.
- Very low blood pressure can result from higher doses.
- Blood problems and rashes have been reported in humans taking benazepril, but this side effect is very rare.

How Should It Be Given?

- The successful outcome of your animal's treatment with this medication depends upon your commitment and ability to administer it exactly as the veterinarian has prescribed. Please do not skip doses or stop giving the medication. If you have difficulty giving doses consult your veterinarian or pharmacist who can offer administration techniques or change the dosage form to a type of medication that may be more acceptable to you and your animal.
- If you miss a dose of this medication you should give it as soon as you remember it, but if it is within a few hours of the regularly scheduled dose, wait and give it at the regular time. Do not double a dose as this can be toxic to your pet.
- Some other drugs can interact with this medication so tell your veterinarian about any drugs or foods that you currently give your animal. Do not give new foods or medications without first asking your veterinarian.
- **Dogs and Cats**: Dogs and cats usually receive benazepril orally once daily.
- **Horses**: Benazepril has been rarely used in horses and is considered a Class 4 drug by the Association of Racing Commissioners International.

What Other Information Is Important About This Medication?

- Benazepril should be stored in a tight, light resistant, childproof container away from all children and other household pets.

Bethanechol

Urecholine® is another name for this medication.

How Is This Medication Useful?

- Bethanechol is used to cause constriction of the bladder to help animals that have difficulty urinating.

Are There Conditions or Times When Its Use Might Cause More Harm Than Good?

- Bethanechol should not be used in animals who have stones blocking their bladder, or if they have had recent bladder surgery.
- This drug should also not be used in animals that have a stomach obstruction.
- If your animal has any of the above conditions, talk to your veterinarian about the potential risks of using the medication versus the benefits that it might have.

What Side Effects Can Be Seen With Its Use?

- When given orally, bethanechol can cause vomiting, diarrhea, lack of appetite and increased drooling. In very high oral doses or after injection, bethanechol may cause heart and breathing problems.
- In horses, bethanechol may cause watery eyes, drooling and stomach cramps.

How Should It Be Given?

- Bethanechol should be given on an empty stomach unless otherwise instructed. The successful outcome of your animal's treatment with this medication depends upon your commitment and ability to administer it exactly as the veterinarian has prescribed. Please do not skip doses or stop giving the medication. If you have difficulty giving doses consult your veterinarian or pharmacist who can offer administration techniques or change the dosage form to a type of medication that may be more acceptable to you and your animal.

- If you miss a dose of this medication you should give it as soon as you remember it, but if it is within a few hours of the regularly scheduled dose, wait and give it at the regular time. Do not double a dose as this can be toxic to your pet.
- Some other drugs can interact with this medication so tell your veterinarian about any drugs or foods that you currently give your animal. Do not give new foods or medications without first asking your veterinarian.
- **Dogs and Cats**: Dogs and cats usually receive this drug orally three times daily.
- **Horses**: This drug is not usually given to horses but when used it is given as an injection under the skin. Bethanechol is considered a Class 4 drug by the Association of Racing Commissioners International.

What Other Information Is Important About This Medication?

- Bethanechol should be stored in a tight, light resistant, childproof container away from all children and other household pets.
- Bethanechol normally has a slight fishy odor; this does not mean that the drug has gone bad.

VETERINARY DRUG HANDBOOK-Client Information Edition
Permission to photocopy for individual clients granted by Gigi Davidson and Donald C. Plumb © 2003

Bisacodyl

Modane® and Dulcolax® are other names for this medication.

How Is This Medication Useful?

- Bisacodyl is used as a stimulant laxative in dogs and cats.

Are There Conditions or Times When Its Use Might Cause More Harm Than Good?

- Bisacodyl should not be used in animals that have an obstruction in their gastrointestinal tract. Those animals who have recently undergone surgery of the stomach or intestines should not receive bisacodyl as stimulation from this drug may cause the incision to come apart.
- This drug may cause other drugs to go through the intestines so fast that they will not be properly absorbed. Do not give this drug within two hours of other drugs.
- Chronic use of bisacodyl may cause the intestines to become flaccid and prevent your animal from efficiently eliminating feces. Do not give this medication without your veterinarian's recommendation.
- If your animal has any of the above conditions, talk to your veterinarian about the potential risks of using the medication versus the benefits that it might have.

What Side Effects Can Be Seen With Its Use?

- Stomach pain and intestinal cramping are most commonly reported from bisacodyl.
- Diarrhea may also result from use of biascodyl.
- Do not give milk or antacids within one hour of bisacodyl as these agents will dissolve the protective coating resulting in destruction of the drug before it reaches its target in the gastrointestinal tract.

How Should It Be Given?

- Bisacodyl can be given orally or in the rectum. Do not crush the tablets or allow your animal to chew them or severe stomach cramps and pain may result. The successful outcome of your animal's treatment with this medication depends upon your commitment and ability to administer it exactly as the veterinarian has prescribed. Please do not skip doses or stop giving the medication. If you have difficulty giving doses consult your veterinarian or pharmacist who can offer administration techniques or change the dosage form to a type of medication that may be more acceptable to you and your animal.
- If you miss a dose of this medication you should give it as soon as you remember it, but if it is within a few hours of the regularly scheduled dose, wait and give it at the regular time. Do not double a dose as this can be toxic to your pet.
- Some other drugs can interact with this medication so tell your veterinarian about any drugs or foods that you currently give your animal. Do not give new foods or medications without first asking your veterinarian.
- **Dogs and Cats**: Dogs and cats usually receive this drug as an oral tablet or as an enema solution. Bisacodyl is usually only given for short periods of time.
- **Horses**: Bisacodyl is not usually given to horses due to an increased risk of colic.

What Other Information Is Important About This Medication?

- Bisacodyl should be stored in a tight, light resistant, childproof container away from all children and other household pets.
- Tablets should not be crushed or chewed as intense stomach cramping and pain may result.

Bismuth Subsalicylate

Pepto Bismol®, Bismusal®, Bismukote®, and Corrective Mixture® are other names for this medication.

How Is This Medication Useful?

- Bismuth subsalicylate is used to treat diarrhea in animals and may also be used as part of a multidrug therapy to get rid of a gastrointestinal bacteria called Helicobacter.

Are There Conditions or Times When Its Use Might Cause More Harm Than Good?

- Because salicylate is in the same family as aspirin, bismuth subsalicylate should not be used in patients who are allergic to or sensitive to aspirin.
- Bismuth subsalicylate should not be used in patients who have bleeding problems.
- Because cats are very sensitive to aspirin and can easily die from overdoses, this drug should probably not be used in cats.
- This drug may cause gastrointestinal obstruction in some patients.
- This drug should not be used at the same time as aspirin due to the increased risk of adverse effects.
- Bismuth subsalicylate can inactivate many drugs and should not be given within 2 hours of any other drug.
- Bismuth subsalicylate can cause false results in urine glucose testing and glucose fluctuations may need to be monitored by blood testing while on salicylates.
- Bismuth subsalicylate will interefere with the accuracy of gastrointestinal x-rays.
- If your animal has any of the above conditions, talk to your veterinarian about the potential risks of using the medication versus the benefits that it might have.

What Side Effects Can Be Seen With Its Use?

- Bismuth subsalicylate may result in constipation.
- The salicylate component of bismuth subsalicylate may be absorbed from the gastrointestinal tract and cause bleeding problems.

How Should It Be Given?

- Shake this medication very well prior to administering.
- The successful outcome of your animal's treatment with this medication depends upon your commitment and ability to administer it exactly as the veterinarian has prescribed. Please do not skip doses or stop giving the medication. If you have difficulty giving doses consult your veterinarian or pharmacist who can offer administration techniques or change the dosage form to a type of medication that may be more acceptable to you and your animal.
- If you miss a dose of this medication you should give it as soon as you remember it, but if it is within a few hours of the regularly scheduled dose, wait and give it at the regular time. Do not double a dose as this can be toxic to your pet.
- Some other drugs can interact with this medication so tell your veterinarian about any drugs or foods that you currently give your animal. Do not give new foods or medications without first asking your veterinarian. You should not give any other drugs within two hours of this medication unless otherwise instructed by your veterinarian.
- **Dogs and Cats**: Dogs and cats usually receive this drug up to three times daily orally for treating diarrhea and an infection called Helicobacter.
- **Horses**: Horses usually receive this drug orally three to fours times daily for diarrhea. The Association of Racing Commissioners International considers this drug to be a Class 4 drug.

What Other Information Is Important About This Medication?

- Bismuth subsalicylate should be stored in a tight, light resistant, childproof container away from all children and other household pets.
- Bismuth subsalicylate suspensions should be shaken well prior to use to ensure that adequate doses of medication are given.

Bromides
Potassium Bromide
Sodium Bromide

KBr is another name for this medication.

How Is This Medication Useful?
- Potassium bromide or sodium bromide are used to treat dogs with epilepsy.

Are There Conditions or Times When Its Use Might Cause More Harm Than Good?
- Bromides must be eliminated from the body by the kidneys. Animals with kidney disease may have problems with this drug.
- Human infants have suffered growth retardation when born to mothers who took bromides. Potassium bromide should probably not be used in pregnant or nursing mothers unless the benefit of use outweighs the risk of adverse effects.
- The intake of chloride will have to be very carefully controlled while your animal is on this drug. Do not give your animal any salty treats and always check with your veterinarian before giving new foods or snacks while on this medication.
- If your animal has any of the above conditions, talk to your veterinarian about the potential risks of using the medication versus the benefits that it might have.

What Side Effects Can Be Seen With Its Use?
- Bromides can cause drowsiness for up to three weeks after starting the drug. Most dogs will eventually become tolerant of this effect and will not remain drowsy during further therapy.
- This drug is irritating to the gastrointestinal tract and can cause vomiting. Giving with food may decrease this effect. Preferably give the drug in food in an elevated food bowl as this will help reduce the chances that if the dog vomits, it will not be inhaled into the lungs.
- Cats can develop a lower respiratory condition (like asthma) when taking potassium bromide. If potassium bromide is used in your cat, you should watch it very closely for signs of coughing and difficulty breathing.
- This drug can also cause excessive thirst, excessive drinking and excessive urination, and has also been known to cause lack of appetite, vomiting and constipation.
- Rashes have been reported in both humans and dogs receiving this drug.

How Should It Be Given?
- Potassium bromide should be given with food fed from elevated food bowls. If capsules are given, care must be taken to ensure that the animal completely swallows the capsules and that sufficient food or water is given to carry the capsule all the way to the stomach. Capsules getting "stuck" between the mouth and stomach can cause severe irritation and damage to the throat and esophagus.
- When you first start bromide therapy, your veterinarian may instruct you to give doses that are 5 times the normal dose. This is to get bromide into your animal's bloodstream more quickly. This is called "loading". You should follow your veterinarian's instructions very carefully during this period to achieve maximum response to therapy as well as to avoid any side effects. If your animal develops any muscle pain or twitching, behavior change or uneven pupils, during this loading period, you should contact your veterinarian immediately.
- The successful outcome of your animal's treatment with this medication depends upon your commitment and ability to administer it exactly as the veterinarian has prescribed. Please do not skip doses or stop giving the medication. If you have difficulty giving doses consult your veterinarian or pharmacist who can offer administration techniques or change the dosage form to a type of medication that may be more acceptable to you and your animal.
- If you miss a dose of this medication you should give it as soon as you remember it, but if it is within a few hours of the regularly scheduled dose, wait and give it at the regular time. Do not double a dose as this can be toxic to your pet.
- Some other drugs can interact with this medication so tell your veterinarian about any drugs or foods that you currently give your animal. Do not give new foods or medications without first asking your veterinarian.
- **Dogs and Cats**: Dogs usually receive this drug orally once daily for life. It can be given as a capsule, a liquid or a chewable treat.
- **Horses**: This drug is not used in horses.

What Other Information Is Important About This Medication?
- Bromides should be stored in a tight, light resistant, childproof container away from all children and other household pets.

Bromocriptine

Parlodel® is another name for this medication.

How Is This Medication Useful?

- Bromocriptine has been used to treat Cushing's disease in horses and some dogs and has also been used to eliminate false pregnancies in dogs.

Are There Conditions or Times When Its Use Might Cause More Harm Than Good?

- Bromocriptine should not be used in patients that have high blood pressure.
- Animals with liver disease will have difficulty eliminating bromocriptine from their bodies and are more at risk for toxicity.
- Bromocriptine should not be used in pregnant animals and, as it stops the flow of milk, should not be used in nursing mothers.
- If your animal has any of the above conditions, talk to your veterinarian about the potential risks of using the medication versus the benefits that it might have.

What Side Effects Can Be Seen With Its Use?

- Typical adverse effects from bromocriptine include nausea and vomiting. Giving the medication with food may reduce these effects.
- Bromocriptine also causes fatigue, drowsiness and lowers blood pressure.

How Should It Be Given?

- Bromocriptine should be given with food to decrease the risk of nausea and vomiting. The successful outcome of your animal's treatment with this medication depends upon your commitment and ability to administer it exactly as the veterinarian has prescribed. Please do not skip doses or stop giving the medication. If you have difficulty giving doses consult your veterinarian or pharmacist who can offer administration techniques or change the dosage form to a type of medication that may be more acceptable to you and your animal.

- If you miss a dose of this medication you should give it as soon as you remember it, but if it is within a few hours of the regularly scheduled dose, wait and give it at the regular time. Do not double a dose as this can be toxic to your pet.
- Some other drugs can interact with this medication so tell your veterinarian about any drugs or foods that you currently give your animal. Do not give new foods or medications without first asking your veterinarian.
- **Dogs and Cats**: Dogs will receive this drug orally once daily with food for 1-2 weeks to end symptoms of false pregnancy.
- **Horses**: Horses will receive this drug as an injection twice daily to treat pituitary adenoma (Cushing's Disease). It must not be used in performing horses, however, as the Association of Racing Commissioners International has declared it a Class 2 drug.

What Other Information Is Important About This Medication?

- Bromocriptine should be stored in a tight, light resistant, childproof container away from all children and other household pets.

VETERINARY DRUG HANDBOOK-Client Information Edition
Permission to photocopy for individual clients granted by Gigi Davidson and Donald C. Plumb © 2003

Buprenorphine

Buprenex® is another name for this medication.

How Is This Medication Useful?
- Buprenorphine is used as a pain medication for dogs and cats.

Are There Conditions or Times When Its Use Might Cause More Harm Than Good?
- Buprenorphine must be eliminated by the kidneys and should be used carefully in animals with kidney disease.
- The liver is also responsible for removing buprenorphine from the body and this drug should be used carefully in animals with liver disease.
- Buprenorphine can depress breathing ability and should be used very carefully in animals that have lung injury or lung disease.
- Certain flea collars and dips containing amitraz (an MAO inhibitor) should not be worn or used within 14 days of buprenorphine as this combination may cause a dangerous rise in body temperature and blood pressure. Aged cheese can also cause this effect, so make sure that your pets do not get into any aged cheese while on this drug.
- Other pain relievers may accentuate the side effects of buprenorphine. Do not administer any other pain relievers to your pet without the recommendation from your veterinarian.
- If your animal has any of the above conditions, talk to your veterinarian about the potential risks of using the medication versus the benefits that it might have.

What Side Effects Can Be Seen With Its Use?
- Sedation is the most commonly experienced side effect.
- Rarely, depression of breathing to the point of respiratory distress has occurred.

How Should It Be Given?
- Buprenorphine injection is usually given to cats orally up to three times daily as needed for pain. The medication should be squirted just under the cat's tongue or in the cheek pouch for maximal effect. The doses are very small for this potent drug, so be sure that you are giving the exact amount that your veterinarian has prescribed.
- The successful outcome of your animal's treatment with this medication depends upon your commitment and ability to administer it exactly as the veterinarian has prescribed. Please do not skip doses or stop giving the medication. If you have difficulty giving doses consult your veterinarian or pharmacist who can offer administration techniques or change the dosage form to a type of medication that may be more acceptable to you and your animal.
- If you miss a dose of this medication you should give it as soon as you remember it, but if it is within a few hours of the regularly scheduled dose, wait and give it at the regular time. Do not double a dose as this can be toxic to your pet.
- Some other drugs can interact with this medication so tell your veterinarian about any drugs or foods that you currently give your animal. Do not give new foods or medications without first asking your veterinarian.
- **Dogs and Cats**: Buprenorphine is usually given orally to dogs and cats up to three times daily for relief of pain. Do not give your pet aged cheese or use tick collars while on this drug.
- **Horses**: Horses may rarely receive buprenorphine for pain relief as an injection. Buprenorphine should not be used in performance horses as the Association of Racing Commissioners International has declared it a Class 2 substance.

What Other Information Is Important About This Medication?
- Buprenorphine should be stored in a tight, light resistant, childproof container away from all children and other household pets.
- Buprenorphine is a controlled substance and should not be given to anyone other than the animal for whom it was prescribed.
- Prescriptions can only be refilled up to 5 times within 6 months of the original prescription date.

Buspirone

Buspar® is another name for this medication.

How Is This Medication Useful?

- Buspirone reduces anxiety and is used to treat behavior problems in your pet.

Are There Conditions or Times When Its Use Might Cause More Harm Than Good?

- Buspirone is removed from the body by the kidneys and liver and should be used carefully in animals with kidney or liver disease.
- After giving this medication for a while, you should not stop it suddenly or the fears and bad behaviors may return.
- Some flea and tick products will cause buspirone to make your pet become very sick. You should tell your veterinarian about all flea products and collars that you use prior to giving this medication.
- Buspirone has not caused problems in pregnant laboratory animals, but should only be used with caution if your pet is pregnant.
- If your animal has any of the above conditions, talk to your veterinarian about the potential risks of using the medication versus the benefits that it might have.

What Side Effects Can Be Seen With Its Use?

- Buspirone does not generally cause any side effects, but can cause a fast heartbeat, dizziness, an upset stomach, headaches and a lack of appetite.
- Too much buspirone can cause your pet to be very drowsy and have constricted pupils. If you notice these symptoms, you should contact your veterinarian immediately.

How Should It Be Given?

- The successful outcome of your animal's treatment with this medication depends upon your commitment and ability to administer it exactly as the veterinarian has prescribed. Please do not skip doses or stop giving the medication. If you have difficulty giving doses consult your veterinarian or pharmacist who can offer administration techniques or change the dosage form to a type of medication that may be more acceptable to you and your animal.

- Some other drugs can interact with this medication so tell your veterinarian about any drugs or foods that you currently give your animal. Do not give new foods or medications without first asking your veterinarian. Report all flea and tick products used to your veterinarian before giving this drug.
- If you miss a dose of this medication you should give it as soon as you remember it, but if it is within a few hours of the regularly scheduled dose, wait and give it at the regular time. Do not double a dose as this can be toxic to your pet. These animals usually receive this drug orally twice or three times daily with or without food.

What Other Information Is Important About This Medication?

- This medication may take 2-4 weeks before it works and as many as one half of patients treated will start to show behavior problems again while on this therapy.
- Buspirone may cause your cat to become more or less affectionate to you and other household pets during therapy.
- Buspirone tablets should be protected from light and moisture.

Butorphanol Tartrate

Torbugesic®, Torbutrol®, and Stadol® are other names for this medication.

How Is This Medication Useful?
- Butorphanol is used in veterinary medicine as a pain reliever and also as a cough suppressant. It may also be used during chemotherapy to prevent chemotherapy-induced vomiting.

Are There Conditions or Times When Its Use Might Cause More Harm Than Good?
- Butorphanol should not be used in patients with liver disease as the drug cannot be efficiently eliminated and may accumulate to toxic levels.
- Animals with diseases of the lungs that produce lots of mucus should not receive butorphanol as this drug prevents removal of the mucus by coughing.
- Because this drug depresses the brain it should not be used in patients with injuries to the head or those in a coma.
- Butorphanol should be used with caution in animals that have kidney disease.
- Although butorphanol is commonly used to suppress cough, it should be used very carefully in animals that have heartworm disease.
- Although it has not been shown to cause birth defects, the manufacturer recommends that butorphanol not be used in pregnancy.
- If your animal has any of the above conditions, talk to your veterinarian about the potential risks of using the medication versus the benefits that it might have.

What Side Effects Can Be Seen With Its Use?
- The most common side effect from butorphanol is drowsiness.
- Some animals may either become overly sedated or overly excited with butorphanol.
- Higher doses may cause horses to become excited, shake their heads and pace.
- Some dogs and cats experience vomiting, loss of appetite and diarrhea from butorphanol. Others may become constipated.
- This drug may also partially reverse the effects of other pain relievers and tranquilizers. Please tell your veterinarian if you are administering any other drugs to your animal.

How Should It Be Given?
- Butorphanol can be given either as an oral tablet or by injection. This drug comes in many different sized tablets and strengths for injection. Make sure that you are using the correct amount as prescribed by your veterinarian.
- The successful outcome of your animal's treatment with this medication depends upon your commitment and ability to administer it exactly as the veterinarian has prescribed. Please do not skip doses or stop giving the medication. If you have difficulty giving doses consult your veterinarian or pharmacist who can offer administration techniques or change the dosage form to a type of medication that may be more acceptable to you and your animal.
- If you miss a dose of this medication you should give it as soon as you remember it, but if it is within a few hours of the regularly scheduled dose, wait and give it at the regular time. Do not double a dose as this can be toxic to your pet.
- Some other drugs can interact with this medication so tell your veterinarian about any drugs or foods that you currently give your animal. Do not give new foods or medications without first asking your veterinarian.
- **Dogs and Cats**: Dogs and cats receive this drug orally or as an injection up to three times daily. Your veterinarian may give this drug more frequently when your pet is in the veterinary hospital.
- **Horses**: Horses receive this drug as an injection to relieve colic pain or for sedation. The Association of Racing Commissioners International has declared butorphanol to be a Class 2 substance.

What Other Information Is Important About This Medication?
- Butorphanol should be stored in a tight, light resistant, childproof container away from all children and other household pets.
- Butorphanol is a controlled substance and should not be given to anyone other than the animal for whom it was prescribed.
- If your pet is taking it chronically for cough, prescriptions can only be refilled up to 5 times within 6 months of the original prescription date.

Captopril

Capoten® is another name for this medication.

How Is This Medication Useful?
Captopril is used to lower blood pressure and to improve heart function.

Are There Conditions or Times When Its Use Might Cause More Harm Than Good?
- Captopril is eliminated by the kidneys and may become toxic in animals with poor kidney function.
- If your animal has low blood sodium then your veterinarian may decide not to use captopril in your pet.
- If your animal has any of the above conditions, talk to your veterinarian about the potential risks of using the medication versus the benefits that it might have.

What Side Effects Can Be Seen With Its Use?
- If the dose is too high, captopril can cause your pet's blood pressure to become too low. If your pet seems like it is weak or it is fainting, you should call your veterinarian immediately.
- Some animals may vomit and develop diarrhea while taking captopril.
- Because captopril contains sulfur, it may cause rashes or skin reactions, and it may also cause the bone marrow to stop producing blood cells.
- At high doses, captopril can cause the kidneys to fail.

How Should It Be Given?
- Captopril should be given on an empty stomach unless otherwise instructed by your veterinarian.
- The successful outcome of your animal's treatment with this medication depends upon your commitment and ability to administer it exactly as the veterinarian has prescribed. Please do not skip doses or stop giving the medication. If you have difficulty giving doses consult your veterinarian or pharmacist who can offer administration techniques or change the dosage form to a type of medication that may be more acceptable to you and your animal.

- If you miss a dose of this medication you should give it as soon as you remember it, but if it is within a few hours of the regularly scheduled dose, wait and give it at the regular time. Do not double a dose as this can be toxic to your pet.
- Some other drugs can interact with this medication so tell your veterinarian about any drugs or foods that you currently give your animal. Do not give new foods or medications without first asking your veterinarian.
- **Dogs and Cats**: Captopril is usually given orally to dogs and cats three times daily.
- **Horses**: Captopril is not usually given to horses and is considered a Class 3 drug by the Association of Racing Commissioners International.

What Other Information Is Important About This Medication?
- Captopril should be stored in a tight, light resistant, childproof container away from all children and other household pets.
- It is normal for captopril to have a rotten egg, sulfurous smell.
- Owners who are allergic to sulfa drugs should handle this drug with caution.

VETERINARY DRUG HANDBOOK-Client Information Edition
Permission to photocopy for individual clients granted by Gigi Davidson and Donald C. Plumb © 2003

Carnitine

Vitamin Bt, L-carnitine and levocarnitine are other names for this medication.

How Is This Medication Useful?

• Carnitine is an amino acid that is essential to normal heart function. It may be used as a supplement for dogs with heart disease where carnitine is deficient. Carnitine may also protect the heart from adverse effects of certain chemotherapy drugs. Carnitine may be useful in cats with fatty liver syndrome. Carnitine may also be used in treating toxicity from certain epilepsy drugs.

Are There Conditions or Times When Its Use Might Cause More Harm Than Good?

• Some products may contain both L-carnitine as well as another form of the drug, d-carnitine. Do not use d-carnitine as this will block the effects of l-carnitine and your pet's condition may worsen.
• Usual carnitine doses may not work as well in epileptic pets that are taking a drug called valproic acid.
• If your animal has any of the above conditions, talk to your veterinarian about the potential risks of using the medication versus the benefits that it might have.

What Side Effects Can Be Seen With Its Use?

• Side effects are not commonly seen with carnitine use. Higher doses may cause vomiting and diarrhea. Giving carnitine with food may decrease stomach upset.
• Humans taking the drug may have an increase in body odor.

How Should It Be Given?

• The successful outcome of your animal's treatment with this medication depends upon your commitment and ability to administer it exactly as the veterinarian has prescribed. Please do not skip doses or stop giving the medication. If you have difficulty giving doses consult your veterinarian or pharmacist who can offer administration techniques or change the dosage form to a type of medication that may be more acceptable to you and your animal.
• If you miss a dose of this medication you should give it as soon as you remember it, but if it is within a few hours of the regularly scheduled dose, wait and give it at the regular time. Do not double a dose as this can be toxic to your pet.
• Some other drugs can interact with this medication so tell your veterinarian about any drugs or foods that you currently give your animal. Do not give new foods or medications without first asking your veterinarian.
• **Dogs & Cats**: Carnitine is usually given to dogs and cats as a powder mixed in food three times daily.
• **Horses**: Carnitine is not usually given to horses.

What Other Information Is Important About This Medication?

• Carnitine should be stored in a tight, light resistant, childproof container away from all children and other household pets.
• Carnitine is very expensive and may be difficult to find in pharmacies. Carnitine powder purchased from health food stores should be examined to make sure that it does not contain any d-carnitine.

Carprofen

Rimadyl® is another name for this medication.

How Is This Medication Useful?

- Carprofen is used in dogs to treat pain and inflammation, due to osteoarthritis or after surgery or injuries. Carprofen is commonly known as an "NSAID" (non-steroidal anti-inflammatory drug).
- Dogs often show improvement very quickly after receiving this drug.

Are There Conditions or Times When Its Use Might Cause More Harm Than Good?

- Carprofen should not be used in animals who are allergic to it or severely allergic to other drugs like it.
- Use this drug very cautiously, if at all, if your dog has active stomach or gastrointestinal ulcers or has had these kinds of ulcers in the past. Carprofen may make these ulcers worse or reappear.
- Speak with your veterinarian if your dog is taking any of the following medications: Other anti-inflammatory drugs such as aspirin or corticosteroids (e.g., prednisone, methylprednisolone, dexamethasone); furosemide (Lasix®), digoxin, methotrexate, sulfa drugs or oral antidiabetic drugs.
- If your animal has or has had heart, kidney or liver problems, talk to your veterinarian about the risks of giving your dog carprofen.
- It is not known if carprofen is safe to give pregnant, lactating or breeding dogs. Talk to your veterinarian before using this drug in those animals.

What Side Effects Can Be Seen With Its Use?

- Carprofen is safe to use in the vast majority of dogs, and the risk of side effects occurring appear to be less than 1%. But rarely, serious side effects and sometimes death have been noted.
- The most commonly reported side effects in dogs taking carprofen are usually related to the gastrointestinal system. This may present as decreased appetite, vomiting (including blood in the vomit), diarrhea, or blood in the stools. If you note any of these, contact your veterinarian.
- Carprofen may also affect the kidneys or the liver. Tell your veterinarian immediately if your dog's water intake or urinary habits have changed or if you see yellowing of the gums, skin or white of the eyes.

- Also immediately contact your veterinarian if your dog is lethargic (lacks energy), is uncoordinated, has seizures or exhibits changes in behavior.

How Should It Be Given?

- The successful outcome of your animal's treatment with this medication depends upon your commitment and ability to administer it exactly as the veterinarian has prescribed. Please do not skip doses or stop giving the medication. If you have difficulty giving doses consult your veterinarian or pharmacist who can offer administration techniques or change the dosage form to a type of medication that may be more acceptable to you and your animal.
- Some other drugs can interact with this medication so tell your veterinarian about any drugs or foods that you currently give your animal. Do not give new foods or medications without first asking your veterinarian.
- **Dogs:** Dogs usually receive this medication once or twice a day by mouth.
- If you are giving this drug every 12 hours (twice a day) and you miss a dose of this medication, you should give it either as soon as you remember or with the next dose.
- If giving this drug once daily and you miss a dose and it is within 12 hours of when you should have given it, give the dose. Otherwise skip this dose and give the next dose at the regular time. Do not double a dose when giving it once a day as this can be toxic to your dog.
- This medication may be given with food or alone, giving with food might reduce the chances of stomach problems occurring.

What Other Information Is Important About This Medication?

- Because the chewable formulation of this drug may be very appealing to dogs, be sure to store in a secure area to prevent an accidental overdose.
- Keep the tablets stored in the original prescription vial at room temperature; do not expose them to high heat.
- Keep this medication away from children.
- Carprofen at this time is NOT considered to be safe to use in cats.
- If you have any other questions or concerns about this medication, be sure to talk to your veterinarian.

Cefadroxil

Cefa-Tabs® Cefa-Drops® and Duricef® are other names for this medication.

How Is This Medication Useful?

- Cefadroxil is an antibiotic that is given orally to treat infections in animals.

Are There Conditions or Times When Its Use Might Cause More Harm Than Good?

- Animals that are allergic to penicillin or penicillin-like drugs should not receive cefadroxil.
- Cefadroxil must be eliminated from the body by the kidneys, and the dose must be lowered in animals with kidney failure.
- Cefadroxil and other cephalosporins may cause seizures in epileptic animals and should be used with caution in these animals.
- Cefadroxil may cross into the womb and should probably not be used in pregnant animals.
- Cefadroxil may cause false positive results in certain kinds of dip sticks used to test the urine of diabetic animals.
- You should always give all of the medication as directed by your veterinarian. If the entire course of treatment is not finished, the germ causing the infection may become stronger than the antibiotics and cause a worsening infection.
- If your animal has any of the above conditions, talk to your veterinarian about the potential risks of using the medication versus the benefits that it might have.

What Side Effects Can Be Seen With Its Use?

- Cefadroxil does not usually cause side effects, but some animals may experience stomach upset, vomiting and diarrhea. Giving cefadroxil with food may alleviate this effect.
- At extremely high doses, cefadroxil can cause damage to the kidneys as well as cause the bone marrow to stop producing blood cells.
- Cefadroxil should be given on an empty stomach unless your pet experiences stomach upset. Once stomach upset occurs, your veterinarian may recommend that you give cefadroxil with food.

How Should It Be Given?

- The successful outcome of your animal's treatment with this medication depends upon your commitment and ability to administer it exactly as the veterinarian has prescribed. Please do not skip doses or stop giving the medication. If you have difficulty giving doses consult your veterinarian or pharmacist who can offer administration techniques or change the dosage form to a type of medication that may be more acceptable to you and your animal.
- If you miss a dose of this medication you should give it as soon as you remember it, but if it is within a few hours of the regularly scheduled dose, wait and give it at the regular time. Do not double a dose as this can be toxic to your pet.
- Some other drugs can interact with this medication so tell your veterinarian about any drugs or foods that you currently give your animal. Do not give new foods or medications without first asking your veterinarian.
- **Dogs & Cat**s: Dogs and cats usually receive this medication as a tablet or a liquid once or twice daily.
- **Horses**: Horses should not receive this medication orally as it may cause life-threatening diarrhea or colic.

What Other Information Is Important About This Medication?

- Cefadroxil should be stored in a tight, light resistant, childproof container away from all children and other household pets. Liquids should be stored in the refrigerator for no more than 14 days and shaken well before use.
- It is normal for cefadroxil to have a sulfurous smell, almost like that of cat urine.
- Pet owners who are allergic to penicillin or penicillin-like drugs should handle this drug with extreme caution.

Cefixime

Suprax® is another name for this medication.

How Is This Medication Useful?

- Cefixime is a powerful, broad-spectrum antibiotic that is used to treat serious infections that do not respond to other antibiotics.

Are There Conditions or Times When Its Use Might Cause More Harm Than Good?

- Animals that are allergic to penicillin or penicillin-like drugs should probably not receive cefixime.
- Cefixime is eliminated by the kidneys and the dose must be reduced in animals with kidney damage.
- Cefixime and other cephalosporins may precipitate seizures and should be used with caution in epileptic animals.
- You should always give all of the medication as directed by your veterinarian. If the entire course of treatment is not finished, the germ causing the infection may become stronger than the antibiotics and cause a worsening infection.
- If your animal has any of the above conditions, talk to your veterinarian about the potential risks of using the medication versus the benefits that it might have.

What Side Effects Can Be Seen With Its Use?

- Cefixime does not usually cause any side effects, but some animals may experience stomach upset, vomiting or diarrhea. Giving cefixime with food may decrease this effect.
- Some animals may experience rashes from cefixime.
- Cefixime may cause a false positive when used with some brands of dip sticks used to check for sugar in the urine of diabetic animals.

How Should It Be Given?

- Cefixime can be given with or without food. The successful outcome of your animal's treatment with this medication depends upon your commitment and ability to administer it exactly as the veterinarian has prescribed. Please do not skip doses or stop giving the medication. If you have difficulty giving doses consult your veterinarian or pharmacist who can offer administration techniques or change the dosage form to a type of medication that may be more acceptable to you and your animal.
- If you miss a dose of this medication you should give it as soon as you remember it, but if it is within a few hours of the regularly scheduled dose, wait and give it at the regular time. Do not double a dose as this can be toxic to your pet.
- Some other drugs can interact with this medication so tell your veterinarian about any drugs or foods that you currently give your animal. Do not give new foods or medications without first asking your veterinarian.
- **Dogs and Cats**: Dogs and cats usually receive this medication orally as tablets or as a liquid once or twice daily.
- **Horses**: Horses should not receive this medication orally as it may cause a life-threatening diarrhea or colic.

What Other Information Is Important About This Medication?

- Cefixime should be stored in a tight, light resistant, childproof container away from all children and other household pets. Liquids can be stored in or out of the refrigerator but should be discarded after 14 days. Liquids should be shaken well before use.

VETERINARY DRUG HANDBOOK-Client Information Edition
Permission to photocopy for individual clients granted by Gigi Davidson and Donald C. Plumb © 2003

Cephalexin

Keflex®, Keftab® and Biocef® are other names for this medication.

How Is This Medication Useful?

- Cephalexin is an antibiotic of the cephalosporin class given orally to treat infections.

Are There Conditions or Times When Its Use Might Cause More Harm Than Good?

- Animals that are allergic to penicillin or penicillin-like drugs should not take cephalexin.
- Cephalexin and other cephalosporins must be eliminated by the kidneys. Animals with kidney failure may receive a lower dose of the drug.
- Cephalexin and other cephalosporins can cause seizures in epileptic patients and should be used with caution in these animals.
- Cephalosporins are known to cross into the womb and should be used with caution in pregnant animals.
- You should always give all of the medication as directed by your veterinarian. If the entire course of treatment is not finished, the germ causing the infection may become stronger than the antibiotics and cause a worsening infection.
- If your animal has any of the above conditions, talk to your veterinarian about the potential risks of using the medication versus the benefits that it might have.

What Side Effects Can Be Seen With Its Use?

- Cephalosporin does not usually cause side effects, however some animals will experience stomach upset, vomiting and diarrhea. Giving cephalexin with food may help reduce this effect.
- Some dogs receiving cephalexin have experienced excessive salivation, panting and excitability.
- Cats have experienced vomiting and fever. Fever in a cat is a temperature of greater than 103°F.
- Cephalexin in very high doses can cause damage to the kidneys.
- Some animals will experience rashes from cephalexin.
- Cephalexin may cause a false positive when used with some brands of dip sticks used to check for sugar in the urine of diabetic animals.

How Should It Be Given?

- The successful outcome of your animal's treatment with this medication depends upon your commitment and ability to administer it exactly as the veterinarian has prescribed. Please do not skip doses or stop giving the medication. If you have difficulty giving doses consult your veterinarian or pharmacist who can offer administration techniques or change the dosage form to a type of medication that may be more acceptable to you and your animal.
- If you miss a dose of this medication you should give it as soon as you remember it, but if it is within a few hours of the regularly scheduled dose, wait and give it at the regular time. Do not double a dose as this can be toxic to your pet.
- Some other drugs can interact with this medication so tell your veterinarian about any drugs or foods that you currently give your animal. Do not give new foods or medications without first asking your veterinarian.
- **Dogs and Cats**: Dogs and cats usually receive cephalexin orally as a capsule, tablet or liquid two to three times daily.
- **Horses**: Horses should not receive oral cephalexin as this may cause a life-threatening diarrhea or colic.

What Other Information Is Important About This Medication?

- Cephalexin should be stored in a tight, light resistant, childproof container away from all children and other household pets. Oral liquids should be stored in the refrigerator for up to 14 days and shaken well before use.
- Pet owners who are allergic to penicillin and penicillin-like drugs should avoid handling this medication.
- It is normal for cephalexin to have a strong sulfurous odor which may smell like cat urine.

Permission to photocopy for individual clients granted by Gigi Davidson and Donald C. Plumb © 2003

Chlorambucil

Leukeran® is another name for this medication.

How Is This Medication Useful?

- Chlorambucil is a potent drug used to treat certain kinds of cancer. It is also used to suppress the immune system in conditions where this effect is desirable.

Are There Conditions or Times When Its Use Might Cause More Harm Than Good?

- Chlorambucil depresses the function of the bone marrow and should be used with extreme caution in patients who already have bone marrow depression or infection.
- Chlorambucil is known to cause birth defects and should generally not be used in pregnancy. This drug is used to treat life-threatening conditions, however, and you and your veterinarian may decide that use during pregnancy is necessary to save the life of the mother.
- Chlorambucil should not be used in males intended for breeding as permanent infertility may result.
- If your animal has any of the above conditions, talk to your veterinarian about the potential risks of using the medication versus the benefits that it might have.

What Side Effects Can Be Seen With Its Use?

- Chlorambucil most commonly causes bone marrow depression which results in anemias and bleeding disorders. These side effects usually occur about one to two weeks after starting therapy with chlorambucil. If your animal experiences any bruising, bleeding, lethargy (lacking energy), infection or difficulty breathing, you should notify your veterinarian immediately.
- Some breeds of dogs are likely to lose their haircoat after treatment with chlorambucil. Poodles and Kerry Blues are more likely to suffer this effect.
- Liver failure has been reported after use of chlorambucil.
- Breathing problems and gout have also been reported after using chlorambucil.

How Should It Be Given?

- Chlorambucil can also cause side effects in the owner if not handled properly. You should always wear gloves when handling this medication and children should never be allowed to handle this drug.

- The successful outcome of your animal's treatment with this medication depends upon your commitment and ability to administer it exactly as the veterinarian has prescribed. Please do not skip doses or stop giving the medication. If you have difficulty giving doses consult your veterinarian or pharmacist who can offer administration techniques or change the dosage form to a type of medication that may be more acceptable to you and your animal.
- If you miss a dose of this medication you should give it as soon as you remember it, but if it is within a few hours of the regularly scheduled dose, wait and give it at the regular time. Do not double a dose as this can be toxic to your pet.
- Some other drugs can interact with this medication so tell your veterinarian about any drugs or foods that you currently give your animal. Do not give new foods or medications without first asking your veterinarian.
- **Dogs and Cats**: Dogs and cats usually receive this drug orally once every day or every other day to suppress the immune system. For treating cancer, chlorambucil is administered every day to every other day or every 2-3 weeks.
- **Horses**: Horses usually receive this drug orally every 2 weeks for treating cancer.

What Other Information Is Important About This Medication?

- Chlorambucil should be stored in a tight, light resistant, childproof container in the refrigerator out of the reach of all children and other household pets. Chorambucil has a sugar coating on the outside which may make it more appealing to pets and children.
- You should always wear gloves when handling this medication. Children and pregnant women should not come into contact with this drug at all.
- For 48 hours after each dose, you should avoid all contact with your pet's urine, feces, saliva or vomit as there may be enough chlorambucil in these bodily byproducts to cause harm to the owner.

Chloramphenicol

Chloromycetin®, Amphicol®, Duricol® and Viceton® are other names for this medication.

How Is This Medication Useful?

- Chloramphenicol is an antibiotic used for a variety of infections. Rarely, it is very toxic to some humans and because of this, its use is forbidden in animals that will be used for human food.

Are There Conditions or Times When Its Use Might Cause More Harm Than Good?

- Chloramphenicol is banned for use in food-producing animals under penalty of law.
- Because chloramphenicol can cause blood problems, it should not be used in animals who are experiencing anemias or bleeding abnormalities.
- Chloramphenicol is eliminated from the body by the liver and should be avoided in patients who have liver failure. If it must be used, dosages must be adjusted..
- Chloramphenicol should be used with extreme caution, if at all, in baby animals. This drug can cause the blood vessels to fail to properly circulate blood resulting in lack of oxygen to vital organs. This drug is particularly dangerous when used in kittens.
- Because chloramphenicol is secreted in the milk, it should not be given to nursing mothers.
- Chloramphenicol should also not be used in breeding animals, and should not be used in pregnancy due to adverse effects on the bone marrow of the fetus.
- If your animal has any of the above conditions, talk to your veterinarian about the potential risks of using the medication versus the benefits that it might have.

What Side Effects Can Be Seen With Its Use?

- Although it is not as severe as the anemia caused in humans, the development of bone marrow depression is often reported in animals and is related to the size of the dose used.
- Many animals will also experience vomiting, diarrhea, lack of appetite, and depression.
- Chloramphenicol stays in cats bodies longer than any other species and they are therefore more likely to develop adverse effects.
- Chloramphenicol can also severely affect the elimination of other drugs from the body. You should tell your veterinarian about any drugs that your pet is currently taking. Chloramphenicol especially affects drugs used for epilepsy.
- Chloramphenicol can affect your pet's ability to respond properly to a vaccination. If your pet is taking chloramphenicol, all vaccinations should be postponed if possible.

How Should It Be Given?

- Chloramphenicol is very hazardous to some humans in that even very small amounts may cause death in 1 in 10,000 people exposed. You should always wear gloves when handling this drug and children and pregnant women should never handle this drug. If you grind up the tablets to make a powder, you should wear a mask to avoid inhaling this drug.
- The successful outcome of your animal's treatment with this medication depends upon your commitment and ability to administer it exactly as the veterinarian has prescribed. Please do not skip doses or stop giving the medication. If you have difficulty giving doses consult your veterinarian or pharmacist who can offer administration techniques or change the dosage form to a type of medication that may be more acceptable to you and your animal.
- If you miss a dose of this medication you should give it as soon as you remember it, but if it is within a few hours of the regularly scheduled dose, wait and give it at the regular time. Do not double a dose as this can be toxic to your pet.
- Some other drugs can interact with this medication so tell your veterinarian about any drugs or foods that you currently give your animal. Do not give new foods or medications without first asking your veterinarian.
- **Dogs and Cats**: Dogs and cats usually receive this drug orally as a tablet or liquid twice or three times daily.
- **Horses**: Horses usually receive this drug orally four times daily.

What Other Information Is Important About This Medication?

- Chloramphenicol should be stored in a tight, light resistant, childproof container away from all children and other household pets.
- This is an extremely bitter drug and most animals may not accept the drug if the original tablet or capsule is crushed or opened.
- Sunlight breaks down chloramphenicol, so if your pet eliminates outside, you should not be in danger. If your pet has an accident or vomits within 48 hours of a dose, put on gloves before cleaning up the accident and place all waste in a plastic bag and put in the outside trash can.
- Unused chloramphenicol should be returned to your veterinarian or pharmacist for proper disposal.

Chlorpheniramine

Chlortrimeton® and Aller-Chlor® are other names for this medication.

How Is This Medication Useful?

- Chlorpheniramine is primarily used as an antihistamine to stop itching. It is occasionally used as a tranquilizer to calm excited animals.

Are There Conditions or Times When Its Use Might Cause More Harm Than Good?

- Chlorpheniramine should be used with caution in patients with glaucoma or asthma as it may worsen these conditions.
- Chlorpheniramine should also be used with caution in animals that have problems urinating, have prostate enlargement, thyroid problems or heart disease.
- Animals with high blood pressure should not receive this drug.
- Working dogs (*e.g.,* guide dogs, search dogs, hunting dogs, sled dogs, rescue dogs) may become overly sedated and unable to perform their duties while on this drug.
- If your animal has any of the above conditions, talk to your veterinarian about the potential risks of using the medication versus the benefits that it might have.

What Side Effects Can Be Seen With Its Use?

- The most common side effect, which is desirable in most cases, is sleepiness and sedation. Most animals will become tolerant to this effect with time and the sleepiness will wear off.
- Dry mouth and inability to urinate are also possible side effects.
- Cats may become unusually excited while taking this drug.
- Animals receiving chlorpheniramine will have a reduced response to allergy testing. Chlorpheniramine should be stopped at least 4 days before allergy tests are started.

How Should It Be Given?

- The successful outcome of your animal's treatment with this medication depends upon your commitment and ability to administer it exactly as the veterinarian has prescribed. If you have difficulty giving any doses, please do not skip doses or stop giving the medication. Most cats despise the taste of chlorpheniramine and getting cats to accept this drug is a challenge. Consult your veterinarian or pharmacist who can offer administration techniques or change the dosage form to a type of medication that may be more acceptable to you and your animal.
- If you miss a dose of this medication you should give it as soon as you remember it, but if it is within a few hours of the regularly scheduled dose, wait and give it at the regular time. Do not double a dose as this can be toxic to your pet.
- Some other drugs can interact with this medication so tell your veterinarian about any drugs or foods that you currently give your animal. Do not give new foods or medications without first asking your veterinarian.
- **Dogs and Cats**: Dogs and cats usually receive this drug orally two to three times daily as a tablet, capsule or liquid.
- **Horses**: Horses do not usually receive this medication, but if given to performance horses, use is considered Class 4 by the Association of Racing Commissioners International.

What Other Information Is Important About This Medication?

- Chlorpheniramine should be stored in a tight, light resistant, childproof container away from all children and other household pets.
- If you are using a long-acting capsule of chlorpheniramine, you may empty the contents of the capsule over food, but do not allow the beads to dissolve before the pet eats the food.

VETERINARY DRUG HANDBOOK-Client Information Edition
Permission to photocopy for individual clients granted by Gigi Davidson and Donald C. Plumb © 2003

Chlorpromazine

Thorazine® is another name for this medication.

How Is This Medication Useful?

- Chlorpromazine is a member of the phenothiazine drugs and is primarily used to stop vomiting in animals.

Are There Conditions or Times When Its Use Might Cause More Harm Than Good?

- Chlorpromazine should be used very carefully in animals with liver disease, heart disease or general lack of well-being.
- Chlorpromazine can cause the blood pressure to drop severely and should be used carefully in animals with pre-existing low blood pressure.
- Chlorpromazine and other phenothiazines have caused seizures in animals who are epileptic or have a history of seizures.
- Chlorpromazine should generally not be given to horses as they may experience agitation, excitement and aggression. Many will have a panic attack. They will also lose their balance, and may injure themselves as well as those humans near them.
- If your animal has any of the above conditions, talk to your veterinarian about the potential risks of using the medication versus the benefits that it might have.

What Side Effects Can Be Seen With Its Use?

- Chlorpromazine and other phenothiazines can cause sedation in all animals.
- Chlorpromazine can cause very low blood pressure and dogs seem to be most likely to suffer from this effect.
- When given to male animals, phenothiazines can cause the penis to protrude and the animal may be unable to retract it for up to 2 hours. Care should be taken to ensure that the animal does not injure its penis while it is protruded.
- Some animals may have an opposite reaction to chlorpromazine and get excited and aggressive.

How Should It Be Given?

- The successful outcome of your animal's treatment with this medication depends upon your commitment and ability to administer it exactly as the veterinarian has prescribed. Please do not skip doses or stop giving the medication. If you have difficulty giving doses consult your veterinarian or pharmacist who can offer administration techniques or change the dosage form to a type of medication that may be more acceptable to you and your animal.
- If you miss a dose of this medication you should give it as soon as you remember it, but if it is within a few hours of the regularly scheduled dose, wait and give it at the regular time. Do not double a dose as this can be toxic to your pet.
- Some other drugs can interact with this medication so tell your veterinarian about any drugs or foods that you currently give your animal. Do not give new foods or medications without first asking your veterinarian.
- **Dogs and Cats**: Dogs and cats usually receive this drug as an injection to stop vomiting.
- **Horses**: This drug should not be used in horses due to the danger to them as well as to humans around them. Chlorpromazine is a Class 2 drug according to the Association of Racing Commissioners International.

What Other Information Is Important About This Medication?

- Chlorpromazine should be stored in a tight, light resistant, childproof container away from all children and other household pets.
- Chlorpromazine will turn yellowish brown upon exposure to light. Discolored solutions should not be used.

Cimetidine

Tagamet® is another name for this medication.

How Is This Medication Useful?

- Cimetidine is used to decrease acid secretion in the stomach and help treat and protect against the formation of ulcers. Cimetidine was the first drug of its kind to reach the market, but its use in veterinary medicine has diminished in recent years. Drugs such as ranitidine or famotidine have fewer drug interactions and dosing is required less often than with cimetidine.

Are There Conditions or Times When Its Use Might Cause More Harm Than Good?

- Cimetidine should be used carefully in animals with blood abnormalities.
- Cimetidine should also be used carefully in animals with liver and kidney disease as the drug is removed from the body by these organs and may accumulate if these organs are not working properly.
- Use cimetidine carefully in older animals.
- Cimetidine can significantly reduce an animal's ability to eliminate several other drugs from the body. Tell your veterinarian about any other drugs you are giving your pet and do not give new drugs without first asking your veterinarian.
- If your animal has any of the above conditions, talk to your veterinarian about the potential risks of using the medication versus the benefits that it might have.

What Side Effects Can Be Seen With Its Use?

- There are few side effects associated with cimetidine in animals, but if your animal shows something abnormal, contact your veterinarian.

How Should It Be Given?

- Preferably cimetidine should be given on an empty stomach as giving with food will cause acid secretion before the drug starts to work. However it is better to give the medication than not to, regardless of feeding status.

- The successful outcome of your animal's treatment with this medication depends upon your commitment and ability to administer it exactly as the veterinarian has prescribed. Please do not skip doses or stop giving the medication. If you have difficulty giving doses consult your veterinarian or pharmacist who can offer administration techniques, change the dosage form or find an alternative medication that may be more acceptable to you and your animal.
- If you miss a dose of this medication you should give it as soon as you remember it, but if it is within a few hours of the regularly scheduled dose, wait and give it at the regular time.
- There are many drugs that can interact with cimetidine. Tell your veterinarian about any drugs or foods that you currently give your animal and do not give new foods or medications without first asking your veterinarian.
- **Dogs and Cats**: Dogs and cats usually receive this drug three to four times a day.
- **Horses**: Foals may receive this drug as an injection ore orally two to four times a day.
- **Ferrets**: May receive this drug orally or by injection 3 times a day.
- **Rabbits, Rodents, Hamsters, Guinea pigs, etc**: May receive this drug two to four times a day.

What Other Information Is Important About This Medication?

- Cimetidine tablets and oral liquid should be stored in a tight, light resistant, childproof container away from all children and other household pets.
- Keep cimetidine products at room temperature.
- Cats particularly do not like the taste of cimetidine liquid and will drool excessively after this medication is given. You can ask your pharmacist about compounding capsules or specially flavored liquids that will make it easier to get your cat to take cimetidine.

Cisapride

Propulsid® is another name for this medication.

How Is This Medication Useful?

- Cisapride stimulates your animal's intestines to move and is useful in treating chronic constipation or other conditions where the gastrointestinal tract has stopped moving food and waste.

Are There Conditions or Times When Its Use Might Cause More Harm Than Good?

- Although this has not been reported in animals, serious drug interactions between antihistamines and antibiotics and cisapride have caused death in people. For this reason, cisapride is no longer available for humans. You should tell your veterinarian about any drugs or other products that your pet is taking.
- Cisapride should not be given to animals who have an immovable obstruction in their gastrointestinal tract as this will worsen the condition.
- Cisapride should be used with caution in animals with heart conditions as cisapride may affect heart rate and beat.
- Cisapride has caused birth defects in laboratory animals and should not be used in pregnant animals.
- Cisapride is removed from the body by the liver and should be used carefully in pets with liver disease.
- If your animal has any of the above conditions, talk to your veterinarian about the potential risks of using the medication versus the benefits that it might have.

What Side Effects Can Be Seen With Its Use?

- The most common side effects are diarrhea and increased bowel activity. Your pet may initially experience some abdominal cramping when cisapride is given.
- Cisapride may also cause your pet to become more excited than usual in higher doses. You should notify your veterinarian immediately if you notice that your pet seems more restless than usual.

How Should It Be Given?

- The successful outcome of your animal's treatment with this medication depends upon your commitment and ability to administer it exactly as the veterinarian has prescribed. Please do not skip doses or stop giving the medication. If you have difficulty giving doses consult your veterinarian or pharmacist who can offer administration techniques or change the dosage form to a type of medication that may be more acceptable to you and your animal.
- Some other drugs can interact with this medication so tell your veterinarian about any drugs or foods that you currently give your animal. Do not give new foods or medications without first asking your veterinarian.
- Cisapride is no longer commercially available and must be compounded by your pharmacist. If you receive a liquid form of cisapride, make sure you shake it well in the container before opening it.
- If you miss a dose of this medication you should give it as soon as you remember it, but if it is within a few hours of the regularly scheduled dose, wait and give it at the regular time. Do not double a dose as this can be toxic to your pet.
- **Dogs and Cats**: These pets usually receive cisapride two to three times daily.

What Other Information Is Important About This Medication?

- Cisapride is no longer commercially available and will have to be compounded by your pharmacist.
- Cisapride should be protected from light and moisture.
- This drug should not be given to any human household members as it can cause fatal side effects in humans who are also receiving certain medications such as antihistamines and antibiotics.

Clemastine

Tavist® and Antihist-1® are other names for this medication.

How Is This Medication Useful?

- Clemastine is used as an antihistamine primarily to stop itching.

Are There Conditions or Times When Its Use Might Cause More Harm Than Good?

- Clemastine should be used with caution in patients with glaucoma or severe heart disease, as it may worsen these conditions.
- Clemastine should also be used with caution in animals that have problems urinating, have prostate enlargement, or have obstructions in the gastrointestinal tract.
- Working dogs (e.g., guide dogs, search dogs, hunting dogs, sled dogs, rescue dogs) may become overly sedated and unable to perform their duties while on this drug.
- If your animal has any of the above conditions, talk to your veterinarian about the potential risks of using the medication versus the benefits that it might have.

What Side Effects Can Be Seen With Its Use?

- The most common side effect, which may be desirable, is sleepiness and sedation. Most animals will become tolerant to this effect with time and the sleepiness will wear off.
- Dry mouth and inability to urinate are also possible side effects.
- Sometimes animals may become unusually excited while taking this drug.
- Animals receiving clemastine will have a reduced response to allergy testing. Clemastine should be stopped at least 4 days before allergy tests are started.

How Should It Be Given?

- The successful outcome of your animal's treatment with this medication depends upon your commitment and ability to administer it exactly as the veterinarian has prescribed. If you have difficulty giving any doses, please do not skip doses or stop giving the medication. Consult your veterinarian or pharmacist who can offer administration techniques or change the dosage form to a type of medication that may be more acceptable to you and your animal.
- If you miss a dose of this medication you should give it as soon as you remember it, but if it is within a few hours of the regularly scheduled dose, wait and give it at the regular time. Do not double a dose as this can be toxic to your pet.
- Some other drugs can interact with this medication so tell your veterinarian about any drugs or foods that you currently give your animal. Do not give new foods or medications without first asking your veterinarian.
- **Dogs and Cats**: Dogs and cats usually receive this drug orally twice daily (every 12 hours) as a tablet or liquid.

What Other Information Is Important About This Medication?

- Clemastine tablets or oral solution should be stored in a tight, light resistant, childproof container away from all children and other household pets.
- Keep clemastine at room temperature.

VETERINARY DRUG HANDBOOK-Client Information Edition
Permission to photocopy for individual clients granted by Gigi Davidson and Donald C. Plumb © 2003

Clenbuterol

Ventipulmin® is another name for this medication.

How Is This Medication Useful?

- Clenbuterol opens up the air passages in the lungs and is used to treat horses with lung diseases.

Are There Conditions or Times When Its Use Might Cause More Harm Than Good?

- Clenbuterol can cause severe side effects in humans such as irregular heart beat and severe muscle tremors. It is illegal to use this drug in any animal that will later be used for food.
- Clenbuterol has strong effects on the heart and should not be used in horses that have heart conditions.
- Clenbuterol should not be used in horses that cannot sweat efficiently.
- Clenbuterol should not be used in pregnant mares who are in the last few months of their pregnancy as it can cause the uterus to contract and expel the baby prematurely.
- Clenbuterol overdoses (more than 2ml/100lbs of body weight) have caused death in horses.
- If your animal has any of the above conditions, talk to your veterinarian about the potential risks of using the medication versus the benefits that it might have.

What Side Effects Can Be Seen With Its Use?

- Clenbuterol causes a fast heartbeat, increased sweating and muscle twitching. These side effects should decrease with time as your horse's body gets used to the effects of clenbuterol. If these side effects continue report them to your veterinarian.
- Many drugs will worsen these side effects so you should tell your veterinarian about any other medications or treatments that you give your horse.

How Should It Be Given?

- The successful outcome of your animal's treatment with this medication depends upon your commitment and ability to administer it exactly as the veterinarian has prescribed. Please do not skip doses or stop giving the medication. If you have difficulty giving doses consult your veterinarian or pharmacist who can offer administration techniques or change the dosage form to a type of medication that may be more acceptable to you and your animal.

- Some other drugs can interact with this medication so tell your veterinarian about any drugs or foods that you currently give your animal. Do not give new foods or medications without first asking your veterinarian.
- If you miss a dose of this medication you should give it as soon as you remember it, but if it is within a few hours of the regularly scheduled dose, wait and give it at the regular time. Do not double a dose as this can be toxic to your animal.
- **Dogs and Cats**: Clenbuterol is not used in dogs and cats.
- **Horses**: Clenbuterol is usually given as an oral liquid twice daily. Your veterinarian may increase the dose every 3 days until an adequate effect is achieved. If your horse does not respond after 15 days, the drug is not likely to work in your horse. Once an effective dose is reached, the therapy usually lasts for one month. Do not continue beyond one month unless directed by your veterinarian. Never adjust the dose on your own. Overdoses (greater than 2ml/100lbs body weight) have caused death in some horses.

What Other Information Is Important About This Medication?

- Clenbuterol is banned for use in racing or show horses during performance times.
- Clenbuterol should be kept well away from children and other household pets.
- Clenbuterol should be stored in the well-closed original container, at room temperature and protected from freezing.

Clindamycin

Antirobe® or Cleocin® are other names for this medication.

How Is This Medication Useful?

- Clindamycin is a type of antibiotic that is used to treat certain types of bacterial infections in dogs, cats and ferrets.
- Clindamycin also can be used to treat infections caused by certain types of parasites called protozoa, including the organism that causes Toxoplasmosis in cats.

Are There Conditions or Times When Its Use Might Cause More Harm Than Good?

- Clindamycin should not be used in **horses, ruminants (cattle, sheep, goats), rabbits, hamsters, or guinea pigs** as it may cause severe diarrhea that can cause death.
- Clindamycin should not be given to animals allergic to it or drugs like it (*e.g.*, lincomycin).
- Animals with severe kidney or liver disease should only receive clindamycin with caution. Your veterinarian may reduce the dosage in your animal if this is the case.
- It is not known if clindamycin is safe to use during pregnancy.
- It should be used cautiously in nursing animals as clindamycin can enter into milk and can cause diarrhea in offspring.
- You should always give all of the medication as directed by your veterinarian. If the entire course of treatment is not finished, the germ causing the infection may become stronger than the antibiotics and cause a worsening infection.
- If your animal has any of the above conditions, talk to your veterinarian about the potential risks of using the medication versus the benefits that it might have.

What Side Effects Can Be Seen With Its Use?

- The most common side effects seen in dogs or cats with orally administered clindamycin are vomiting and loose stools.
- If diarrhea becomes bloody, severe, or lasts for several days contact your veterinarian.
- Allergic reactions are possible, but very rare.

How Should It Be Given?

- The successful outcome of your animal's treatment with this medication depends upon your commitment and ability to administer it exactly as the veterinarian has prescribed. Give this drug for the full course of treatment prescribed by your veterinarian, even if your pet is better or seems cured as bacteria may remain that could make the infection worse.
- Please do not skip doses or stop giving the medication. If you have difficulty giving doses consult your veterinarian or pharmacist who can offer administration techniques or change the dosage form to a type of medication that may be more acceptable to you and your animal.
- If you miss a dose of this medication you should give it as soon as you remember it, but if it is within a few hours of the regularly scheduled dose, wait and give it at the regular time. Do not double a dose as this can be toxic to your pet.
- Because some other drugs interact with this medication, especially other antibiotics, you should tell your veterinarian about any drugs or foods that you currently give your animal. Do not give new foods or medications without first asking your veterinarian.
- **Dogs and Cats**: Dogs and cats usually receive this drug orally once to two times daily as a tablet or liquid. Your veterinarian my also inject this medication.
- **Ferrets**: Ferrets usually receive this drug twice a day.
- **Horses**: Horses should generally not receive this medication as it can cause severe diarrhea.
- **Rabbits, Hamsters, Guinea pigs, Gerbils**: Should not receive this medication as it can cause severe diarrhea and death.

What Other Information Is Important About This Medication?

- Clindamycin should be stored in a tight, light resistant, childproof container away from all children and other household pets.
- This medication may be stored at room temperature.
- If you are using the human-label oral solution (Cleocin® Pediatric), it should be discarded after two weeks.
- It often takes a few days for this medication to reduce the signs of infection in your animal, but if your animal does not show some improvement after several days of treatment, or if their condition gets worse, contact your veterinarian.

VETERINARY DRUG HANDBOOK-Client Information Edition
Permission to photocopy for individual clients granted by Gigi Davidson and Donald C. Plumb © 2003

Clomipramine

Clomicalm® and Anafranil® are other names for this medication.

How Is This Medication Useful?

- Clomipramine is primarily used in dogs to help reduce unwanted behaviors such as dominance aggression, separation anxiety, and obsessive-compulsive behaviors such as excessive grooming, pacing, etc.
- It can be used in cats to help reduce unwanted behaviors such as urine marking/spraying, aggression with other cats or people, or compulsive behaviors (grooming, wool-sucking). Dosing tends to be more difficult in cats and they can be more sensitive than dogs to the side effects of this medication.

Are There Conditions or Times When Its Use Might Cause More Harm Than Good?

- Clomipramine should not be used in animals who have had prior sensitivity reactions to it or other drugs like it (e.g., amitriptyline).
- Clomipramine could possibility increase the incidence of seizures in animals with epilepsy.
- It should also be used with caution in animals that have problems urinating, decreased gastrointestinal function, heart disease, liver disease, thyroid disease or glaucoma.
- Clomipramine should not be used in animals who are also receiving drugs known as MAO inhibitors (Mitaban® Dip, Preventic® Flea Collars, Anipryl®, and isoniazid are a few of these drugs). When clomipramine is given with these drugs it can cause serious increases in blood pressure that can cause death. Aged cheese can also cause this effect, so make sure that your pets do not get into any aged cheese while on this drug. If your pet is receiving any of these medications, your veterinarian will ask you to stop giving them for at least 2-5 weeks before he prescribes clomipramine.
- Working dogs (e.g., guide dogs, search dogs, hunting dogs, sled dogs, rescue dogs) may become overly sedated and unable to perform their duties while on this drug.
- If your animal has any of the above conditions, talk to your veterinarian about the potential risks of using the medication versus the benefits that it might have.

What Side Effects Can Be Seen With Its Use?

- The most common side effects in pets include sleepiness, vomiting, and diarrhea. Most animals will become tolerant to these effects with time and the sleepiness should wear off.
- Dry mouth and difficulty with urinating are also possible side effects.
- Cats may be more likely to develop side effects than are dogs.
- Contact your veterinarian if side effects are severe or persist.

How Should It Be Given?

- The successful outcome of your animal's treatment with this medication depends upon your commitment and ability to administer it exactly as the veterinarian has prescribed. If you have difficulty giving any doses, please do not skip doses or stop giving the medication. Consult your veterinarian or pharmacist who can offer administration techniques or change the dosage form to a type of medication that may be more acceptable to you and your animal.
- If you miss a dose of this medication you should give it as soon as you remember it, but if it is within a few hours of the regularly scheduled dose, wait and give it at the regular time. Do not double a dose as this can be toxic to your pet.
- Some other drugs can interact with this medication so tell your veterinarian about any drugs or foods that you currently give your animal. Do not give new foods or medications without first asking your veterinarian.
- **Dogs and Cats**: Dogs and cats usually receive this drug orally one to two times daily as tablets or capsules. Do not give your pet aged cheese or use tick collars while on this drug.

What Other Information Is Important About This Medication?

- Clomipramine should be stored in a tight, light resistant, childproof container away from all children and other household pets.
- Clomipramine should be stored at room temperature.

Codeine

How Is This Medication Useful?

- Codeine is an opiate narcotic that is useful to treat moderate pain, cough and diarrhea primarily in dogs, but also in cats.
- In dogs, pain relief usually begins in about 30 minutes after oral dosing and persists for 4-6 hours.

Are There Conditions or Times When Its Use Might Cause More Harm Than Good?

- Codeine should not be used in animals who are hypersensitive to it or other opiate drugs (morphine, etc).
- Codeine should not be given to animals who are receiving drugs known as MAO inhibitors (Mitaban® Dip, Preventic® Flea Collars, Anipryl®, and isoniazid are a few of these drugs). Aged cheese can also cause this effect, so make sure that your pets do not get into any aged cheese while on this drug.
- It should be used with caution in dogs or cats with thyroid, heart, lung, or adrenal gland diseases.
- Patients with head injuries or old or debilitated animals should receive the drug with caution.
- It must not be used in animals with diarrhea caused by a toxic substance, until that substance has been eliminated.
- Working dogs (e.g., guide dogs, search dogs, hunting dogs, sled dogs, rescue dogs) may become overly sedated and unable to perform their duties while on this drug.
- The combination product that contains codeine and acetaminophen must NOT be used in cats or death may result.
- If your animal has any of the above conditions, talk to your veterinarian about the potential risks of using the medication versus the benefits that it might have.

What Side Effects Can Be Seen With Its Use?

- The most common side effect is sedation. Most animals will become tolerant to this effect with time and the sleepiness will wear off.
- Codeine can cause a variety of gastrointestinal effects, including vomiting, decreased appetite, and constipation.
- Cats may become unusually excited while taking this drug and tremors and seizures have been seen.

How Should It Be Given?

- The successful outcome of your animal's treatment with this medication depends upon your commitment and ability to administer it exactly as the veterinarian has prescribed. If you have difficulty giving any doses, please do not skip doses or stop giving the medication.
- Consult your veterinarian or pharmacist who can offer administration techniques or change the dosage form to a type of medication that may be more acceptable to you and your animal.
- If your veterinarian has prescribed this drug to be used routinely and you miss a dose, you should give it as soon as you remember it, but wait the appropriate amount of time before giving the following doses. Do not double a dose as this can be toxic to your pet.
- Some other drugs can interact with this medication so tell your veterinarian about any drugs or foods that you currently give your animal. Do not give new foods or medications without first asking your veterinarian.
- **Dogs and Cats**: Dogs and cats usually receive this drug orally two to four times daily as a tablet or liquid. Do not give your pet aged cheese or use tick collars while on this drug.
- **Horses**: Horses do not usually receive this medication as it may stop their intestines and cause colic.

What Other Information Is Important About This Medication?

- Codeine is a controlled substance and should not be given to anyone other than the animal for whom it was prescribed. It is in the most restricted category (C-II) when used as a single agent. Your veterinarian will need to write a new prescription each time if this is the form prescribed.
- When prescribed in combination with acetaminophen (not to be used in cats) or aspirin, the medication can be refilled up to 5 times within a 6 month period.
- Codeine tablets or oral solution should be stored at room temperature in a tight, light resistant, childproof container away from all children and other household pets.

VETERINARY DRUG HANDBOOK-Client Information Edition
Permission to photocopy for individual clients granted by Gigi Davidson and Donald C. Plumb © 2003

Cyclophosphamide

Cytoxan® is another name for this medication.

How Is This Medication Useful?

- Cyclophosphamide is used to treat cancer and some diseases that are caused by an overactive immune system.

Are There Conditions or Times When Its Use Might Cause More Harm Than Good?

- Cyclophosphamide is cleared from the body by the liver and kidneys. It should be used very carefully in pets with liver or kidney disease.
- Cyclophosphamide causes the bone marrow to stop producing blood cells and should be used carefully in pets with anemias or those pets on other drugs that suppress the bone marrow. These effects on bone marrow usually occur within 1-2 weeks of treatment and will take about 4 weeks to recover.
- Because cyclophosphamide suppresses the immune system, your pet might be more susceptible to infections while on this medication.
- The effects of cyclophosphamide on the bladder may increase the risk of bladder cancer at a later time.
- Cyclophosphamide may cause birth defects and should not be used during pregnancy.
- If your animal has any of the above conditions, talk to your veterinarian about the potential risks of using the medication versus the benefits that it might have.

What Side Effects Can Be Seen With Its Use?

- Cyclophosphamide decreases the ability of the bone marrow to produce blood cells which may result in anemias and increased risk for infection. If your pet shows signs of lack of energy, weakness, infection, bruising or bleeding you should contact your veterinarian immediately.
- Cyclophosphamide can be toxic to the heart at higher doses. Report any irregular heart beats or rates to your veterinarian.
- Cyclophosphamide may cause stomach upset and can be given with food to reduce this side effect.
- Hair loss is common in those breeds of dogs that are continuously growing hair (*e.g.,* Poodles and Old English Sheepdogs).
- Cyclophosphamide may cause bladder irritation. You should leave lots of clean water for your pet to drink and report any signs of blood in the urine or frequent urination to your veterinarian immediately.

How Should It Be Given?

- The successful outcome of your animal's treatment with this medication depends upon your commitment and ability to administer it exactly as the veterinarian has prescribed. Please do not skip doses or stop giving the medication. If you have difficulty giving doses consult your veterinarian or pharmacist who can offer administration techniques or change the dosage form to a type of medication that may be more acceptable to you and your animal.
- Some other drugs can interact with this medication so tell your veterinarian about any drugs or foods that you currently give your animal. Do not give new foods or medications without first asking your veterinarian.
- If you miss a dose of this medication you should give it as soon as you remember it, but if it is within a few hours of the regularly scheduled dose, wait and give it at the regular time. Do not double a dose as this can be extremely toxic to your pet.
- As cyclophosphamide can cause immune suppression in humans, you should wear gloves and wash hands after giving this medication.
- You should not split or crush these tablets unless directed by your veterinarian as this might result in an unpredictable amount of drug getting into your pet's blood stream.
- **Dogs and Cats:** Dogs and cats usually get this drug orally 4 days out of 7 for 6-8 weeks in a cancer treatment program. You must take your pet back to the veterinarian frequently for very important blood work checkups.

What Other Information Is Important About This Medication?

- Cyclophosphamide tablets should be protected from light and moisture and stored at room temperature. Solutions of cyclophosphamide should be stored in the refrigerator and discarded after 14 days.
- Pet owners who are pregnant, breast-feeding or trying to conceive should not handle this medication.
- Any waste from this animal (feces, urine, saliva) should be cleaned up with gloves for at least 48 hours after the last treatment with cyclophosphamide. Waste should be disposed of in a sealed plastic bag.

Cyclosporine

Neoral®, Sandimmune® and Gengraf® are other names for this medication.

How Is This Medication Useful?

- Cyclosporine is used to slow overactive immune systems. It is used to prevent rejection of transplanted organs, to treat skin and blood conditions that are caused by over active immune systems, and to treat dry eye in dogs. It is also very useful in allowing healing of cracks around the anus (anal fistulas) that do not respond to other treatments.

Are There Conditions or Times When Its Use Might Cause More Harm Than Good?

- Cyclosporine should be used carefully in patients with liver or kidney disease.
- Cyclosporine may keep vaccines from working properly. Your pet should not receive vaccines with live virus while on cyclosporine.
- Cyclosporine causes birth defects and death to the fetus in many animals. It should not be used in pregnancy. Pregnant caregivers should avoid contact with this drug.
- Cyclosporine affects or is affected by many other drugs. You should tell your veterinarian about any drugs that your pet is taking.
- If your animal has any of the above conditions, talk to your veterinarian about the potential risks of using the medication versus its potential benefits.

What Side Effects Can Be Seen With Its Use?

- In dogs, vomiting, diarrhea, and loss of appetite are the most common side effects.
- Cats will lose their appetites when receiving higher doses of cyclosporine.
- Some cats will have increased hair growth while on cyclosporine.
- Cyclosporine can cause overgrowth of the gums.
- Since cyclosporine decreases the power of the immune system, your pet is more susceptible to infection. Watch your pet for signs of infection such as fever (103°-104°F in dogs and cats), tiredness or sneezing, coughing or runny eyes.
- Most animals do not like the taste of cyclosporine and giving gel capsules or flavoring the liquid is recommended.
- In humans, the risk of cancer is sometimes higher in patients who have taken the drug for a long time.

How Should It Be Given?

- Cyclosporine must be given orally on an empty stomach. Animals that vomit cyclosporine may need to have the drug given with food.
- Cyclosporine is very expensive. If your pet needs a high dose of it, the veterinarian may prescribe another drug (erythromycin or ketoconazole) that slows down the removal of cyclosporine from the body. This will allow you to give a lower, and therefore less expensive, dose.
- There are two different kinds of oral liquids of cyclosporine: the microemulsion (Neoral®) and the regular liquid (Sandimmune®). The microemulsion is much stronger and these liquids should not be substituted for each other. Cyclosporine is also inactivated by some kinds of plastics. You should not leave the drug in plastic cups or syringes for long periods of time or it may not work.
- The successful outcome of your animal's treatment with this medication depends upon your commitment and ability to administer it exactly as the veterinarian has prescribed. Please do not skip doses or stop giving the medication. If you have difficulty giving doses consult your veterinarian or pharmacist who can offer administration techniques or change the dosage form to a type of medication that may be more acceptable to you and your animal.
- If you miss a dose of this medication you should give it as soon as you remember it, but if it is within a few hours of the regularly scheduled dose, wait and give it at the regular time. Do not double a dose as this can be toxic to your pet.
- Some other drugs can interact with this medication so tell your veterinarian about any drugs or foods that you currently give your animal. Do not give new foods or medications without first asking your veterinarian.
- **Dogs and Cats**: Dogs and cats usually receive cyclosporine orally once or twice daily on an empty stomach. Food may be given to decrease vomiting if it occurs.
- **Horses**: Horses do not usually receive cyclosporine orally but may receive it as a surgical implant in the eye for certain eye diseases.

What Other Information Is Important About This Medication?

- Cyclosporine should be stored in a tight, light resistant, childproof container away from all children and other household pets.
- You should throw away all open bottles of cyclosporine after they have been opened for 2 months as exposure to air slowly destroys the drug.
- Cyclosporine is an expensive drug therapy. It must also be very carefully monitored so your veterinarian will want you to bring your pet back into the office for very important blood checks to make sure that the drug is not becoming toxic. Be sure to bring your pet back for these very important visits.

Cyproheptadine

Periactin® is another name for this medication.

How Is This Medication Useful?

- Cyproheptadine is an antihistamine used to stop itching in dogs and cats.
- Cyproheptadine can also be used to stimulate appetite in cats.
- Cyproheptadine is used in horses to treat Cushing's disease.

Are There Conditions or Times When Its Use Might Cause More Harm Than Good?

- Cyproheptadine is cleared from the body by the liver and kidneys. It should be used very carefully in pets with liver or kidney disease.
- Cyproheptadine has effects on the smooth muscles of the body. It should be used with caution in pets with prostate problems, glaucoma, problems with urination, bladder stones, heart problems and obstructions in the intestinal tract.
- Cyproheptadine should be used with caution with certain flea and tick collars and dips as these products may cause cyproheptadine to become toxic.
- Cyproheptadine has not been proven to be safe in pregnancy and should probably not be used in pregnant or nursing animals.
- If your animal has any of the above conditions, talk to your veterinarian about the potential risks of using the medication versus the benefits that it might have.

What Side Effects Can Be Seen With Its Use?

- Typically, cyproheptadine will cause sedation, dry mouth, and constipation. It also causes appetite stimulation in cats and is used for this effect in some instances.
- Cats and horses may be stimulated by cyproheptadine.
- Large doses can cause severe effects such as very rapid heartbeat, inability to urinate, fever and possibly seizures and death.

How Should It Be Given?

- The successful outcome of your animal's treatment with this medication depends upon your commitment and ability to administer it exactly as the veterinarian has prescribed. Please do not skip doses or stop giving the medication. If you have difficulty giving doses consult your veterinarian or pharmacist who can offer administration techniques or change the dosage form to a type of medication that may be more acceptable to you and your animal.
- Some other drugs can interact with this medication so tell your veterinarian about any drugs or foods that you currently give your animal. Do not give new foods or medications without first asking your veterinarian.
- If you miss a dose of this medication you should give it as soon as you remember it, but if it is within a few hours of the regularly scheduled dose, wait and give it at the regular time. Do not double a dose as this can be toxic to your pet.
- **Dogs**: Dogs usually receive cyproheptadine orally two or three times daily.
- **Cats**: Cats usually receive cyproheptadine once or twice daily.
- **Horses**: Horses usually receive cyproheptadine once daily but occasionally will receive it twice daily.

What Other Information Is Important About This Medication?

- All products should be protected from light and moisture and should not be frozen. Some compounded solutions may require refrigeration.
- If your animal is scheduled to have allergy tests, you should stop giving cyproheptadine for one week before the tests.

Dalteparin

Fragmin® is another name for this medication.

How Is This Medication Useful?

- Dalteparin is a low molecular weight heparin blood thinner. It is used to prevent blood clots in animals that have had them or are prone to have them. It may also be given before surgery to prevent blood clot formation where excessive clotting might kill the patient.

Are There Conditions or Times When Its Use Might Cause More Harm Than Good?

- Because dalteparin thins the blood, it increases the risk of bleeding. Do not allow your pet to be in situations where it might be injured or cut as it could bleed to death.
- Dalteparin should not be injected into the muscle or into the vein but only under the skin with the very small needle provided by your pharmacist or veterinarian. Most pet owners administer dalteparin with insulin syringes.
- Dalteparin should not be used in animals who have or have had bleeding problems.
- Because dalteparin is collected from pigs, it should not be used in animals that are allergic to pork products. If your animal appears to rub its face on the floor, looks itchy, has swelling of the face or throat, or has trouble breathing, you should take it to the closest veterinarian immediately.
- Dalteparin should be used carefully in animals that have liver or kidney disease.
- Many pain medications (aspirin, acetaminophen, ibuprofen, carprofen, etodolac, deracoxib, etc) also prevent the blood from clotting. Do not use any other medications, even those purchased without a prescription, in your pet without first consulting your veterinarian.
- Dalteparin is not likely to harm unborn babies but should be used in pregnant animals only if the mother's life is in danger.
- If your animal has any of the above conditions, talk to your veterinarian about the potential risks of using the medication versus the benefits that it might have.

What Side Effects Can Be Seen With Its Use?

- Some animals will experience redness and itching at the injection site.
- Some animals will develop a fever from dalteparin. If your cat or dog has a temperature of 103°-104°F you should call your veterinarian for advice.

How Should It Be Given?

- Dalteparin should be injected just under the skin once daily with a very small needle, usually an insulin syringe. Since it is a very potent drug and is given in tiny amounts, you should make sure your pharmacist or veterinarian shows you exactly how much to inject every day.
- Do not shake dalteparin as it may break up the very fragile drug molecule and destroy the effectiveness of the drug.
- It should only be injected just under the skin, not into a vein or into the muscle.
- You should change the injection site daily and not give it too many times in the same spot.
- Don't inject any medication that has changed colors or has specks in it.
- The successful outcome of your animal's treatment with this medication depends upon your commitment and ability to administer it exactly as the veterinarian has prescribed. Please do not skip doses or stop giving the medication. If you have difficulty giving doses consult your veterinarian or pharmacist who can offer administration techniques or change the dosage form to a type of medication that may be more acceptable to you and your animal.
- If you miss a dose of this medication you should give it as soon as you remember it, but if it is within a few hours of the regularly scheduled dose, wait and give it at the regular time. Do not double a dose as this can be toxic to your pet.
- Some other drugs can interact with this medication so tell your veterinarian about any drugs or foods that you currently give your animal. Do not give new foods or medications without first asking your veterinarian.
- **Dogs and Cats**: Dogs and cats usually receive dalteparin as an injection under the skin once daily.

What Other Information Is Important About This Medication?

- Dalteparin should be stored in a tight, light resistant, childproof container away from all children and other household pets.
- It should not be shaken.
- Open vials should be discarded after 30 days.
- Dalteparin is a very expensive therapy.

Deracoxib

Deramaxx® is another name for this medication.

How Is This Medication Useful?

- Deracoxib is useful in reducing pain caused by inflammation especially after a surgical procedure. It is considered to be much safer than aspirin or ibuprofen or acetaminophen.

Are There Conditions or Times When Its Use Might Cause More Harm Than Good?

- Dogs with bleeding problems (*e.g.*, Von Willebrand's Disease) should not take deracoxib as it may stimulate uncontrollable bleeding at higher doses.
- Animals with kidney disease should not take deracoxib as it may worsen the kidney disease.
- Animals with stomach ulcers or bowel disorders should not take deracoxib.
- Cats cannot efficiently eliminate deracoxib and should not receive this drug as it can be toxic to the kidneys.
- Other anti-inflammatory drugs similar to deracoxib have caused birth defects in humans and animals. Deracoxib should probably not be used in pregnant animals.
- If your animal has any of the above conditions, talk to your veterinarian about the potential risks of using the medication versus the benefits that it might have.

What Side Effects Can Be Seen With Its Use?

- Some dogs may develop dry eye (keratoconjunctivitis sicca) after taking drugs like deracoxib. If your dog develops any eye discharge or squinting while taking deracoxib, you should contact your veterinarian immediately.
- Deracoxib is generally free of side effects but may cause vomiting or diarrhea in some animals. You should report these to your veterinarian immediately if they occur.
- Deracoxib at higher doses (two times the normal dose) can cause bleeding in the gastrointestinal tract. Notify your veterinarian immediately if your pet vomits blood or has feces that appear black or tarry.
- Deracoxib and drugs like it may cause liver damage in some animals. You should notify your veterinarian immediately if your pet seems lethargic (lacking energy), vomits, or stops eating.

How Should It Be Given?

- Deracoxib tablets are scored and the dose can be rounded to the nearest ½ tablet. Deracoxib should be given with food to reduce stomach injury or upset.
- The successful outcome of your animal's treatment with this medication depends upon your commitment and ability to administer it exactly as the veterinarian has prescribed. Please do not skip doses or stop giving the medication. If you have difficulty giving doses consult your veterinarian or pharmacist who can offer administration techniques or change the dosage form to a type of medication that may be more acceptable to you and your animal.
- If you miss a dose of this medication you should give it as soon as you remember it, but if it is within a few hours of the regularly scheduled dose, wait and give it at the regular time. Do not double a dose as this can be toxic to your pet.
- Some other drugs can interact with this medication so tell your veterinarian about any drugs or foods that you currently give your animal. Do not give new foods or medications without first asking your veterinarian.
- **Dogs and Cats**: Dogs usually receive deracoxib orally once or twice daily with meals. Cats do not usually receive deracoxib.
- **Horses**: Horses do not usually receive deracoxib, but it is possible that they may receive deracoxib orally once or twice daily.

What Other Information Is Important About This Medication?

- Deracoxib should be stored in a tight, light resistant, childproof container away from all children and other household pets.

Desmopressin

DDAVP® is another name for this medication.

How Is This Medication Useful?

- Desmopressin is a man-made (synthetic) form of the natural hormone vasopressin that controls fluid elimination in the body. Desmopressin is used to control the excessive urination caused by a disease called diabetes insipidus. It is also sometimes used to treat a disease where blood does not clot called Von Willebrand's Disease.

Are There Conditions or Times When Its Use Might Cause More Harm Than Good?

- Desmopressin should not be used in patients who have heart disease or other conditions where they are prone to blood clots.
- Early in desmopressin treatment, your pet may retain too much water in its body. Your veterinarian may ask you to limit the amount of water that your pet drinks.
- Desmopressin should not be used in patients that are allergic to it or to drugs like it. If your pet shows any itching, swelling of the face, tongue or throat, or has difficulty breathing, you should take it to the nearest veterinarian.
- Desmopressin is not likely to harm unborn babies but should probably only be used in pregnant animals if the life of the mother is in danger.
- If your animal has any of the above conditions, talk to your veterinarian about the potential risks of using the medication versus the benefits that it might have.

What Side Effects Can Be Seen With Its Use?

- Desmopressin can cause eye irritation when administered as an eye drop.
- Desmopressin can cause water retention and swelling in the early part of therapy.
- Desmopressin does not have many side effects in animals, but humans have reported headaches, flushing, chills, weakness and dizziness when using desmopressin.

How Should It Be Given?

- Desmopressin should be administered right into the eyelid sac (conjunctival sac) just like an eye drop. Do not touch the tip of the dropper to the eyelid to avoid contamination.
- The successful outcome of your animal's treatment with this medication depends upon your commitment and ability to administer it exactly as the veterinarian has prescribed. Please do not skip doses or stop giving the medication. If you have difficulty giving doses consult your veterinarian or pharmacist who can offer administration techniques or change the dosage form to a type of medication that may be more acceptable to you and your animal.
- If you miss a dose of this medication you should give it as soon as you remember it, but if it is within a few hours of the regularly scheduled dose, wait and give it at the regular time. Do not double a dose as this can be toxic to your pet.
- Some other drugs can interact with this medication so tell your veterinarian about any drugs or foods that you currently give your animal. Do not give new foods or medications without first asking your veterinarian.
- **Dogs and Cats**: Dogs and cats usually receive desmopressin as an eye drop once or twice daily. Some animals may receive the drug orally, but it is usually very much more expensive this way.

What Other Information Is Important About This Medication?

- Desmopressin should be stored in a tight, light resistant, childproof container in the refrigerator away from all children and other household pets.
- Open vials should be discarded after 30 days.
- If your pet starts urinating excessively again, you should contact your veterinarian.

Diazepam

Valium® is another name for this medication.

How Is This Medication Useful?

- Diazepam is used in animals as a sedative, for seizures, and to cause muscle relaxation. It is also used to cause bladder relaxation to allow urination. It has also been given as an antianxiety agent for behavior problems. Given as an injection, it has been used to stimulate appetite in cats.

Are There Conditions or Times When Its Use Might Cause More Harm Than Good?

- Cats may develop a fatal liver problem when given diazepam by mouth. It is not predictable which cats will have this reaction. If your cat already has liver problems, you should not give your cat diazepam orally.
- As diazepam is cleared from the body by the liver and kidneys, it should be used very carefully in pets with liver or kidney disease.
- The effects of sedation can be great with diazepam and it should be used cautiously in large or working animals whose safety or performance may be affected by sedation. Humans working around large animals sedated with diazepam should take care to avoid injury from animals who are unstable or may fall down.
- Diazepam has consistently caused birth defects and should only be used in pregnancy or nursing animals when this risk is acceptable.
- If your animal has any of the above conditions, talk to your veterinarian about the potential risks of using the medication versus the benefits that it might have.

What Side Effects Can Be Seen With Its Use?

- The usual effects are drowsiness and sedation.
- Dogs will sometimes get usually excited from diazepam instead of becoming sedated.
- Horses may experience muscle trembling, weakness and may fall down after receiving higher doses of diazepam.
- Higher doses in any species can cause difficulty breathing.

How Should It Be Given?

- The successful outcome of your animal's treatment with this medication depends upon your commitment and ability to administer it exactly as the veterinarian has prescribed. Please do not skip doses or stop giving the medication. If you have difficulty giving doses consult your veterinarian or pharmacist who can offer administration techniques or change the dosage form to a type of medication that may be more acceptable to you and your animal.
- Some other drugs can interact with this medication so tell your veterinarian about any drugs or foods that you currently give your animal. Do not give new foods or medications without first asking your veterinarian.
- If you miss a dose of this medication you should give it as soon as you remember it, but if it is within a few hours of the regularly scheduled dose, wait and give it at the regular time. Do not double a dose as this can be toxic to your pet.
- **Dogs and Cats**: Dogs and cats usually receive this medication once or twice daily by mouth. If your veterinarian decides to use diazepam by mouth in your cat, you should watch the cat for any signs of the fatal liver problem that oral diazepam can cause. If you cat stops eating or acts depressed, you should stop giving the diazepam and notify your veterinarian immediately. Sometimes your veterinarian will prescribe a solution of diazepam that is inserted into the animal's rectum during a bad seizure. Make sure your veterinarian demonstrates this technique for you so that you will know how to do it if the need arises.
- **Horses**: Horses do not generally receive diazepam outside of the veterinary hospital. Diazepam is banned for use in racing or performance horses during and around show times.

What Other Information Is Important About This Medication?

- Diazepam should be protected from light and moisture and stored at room temperature. Diazepam solutions should not be stored in plastic and should not be mixed with any other drugs.
- Diazepam is a controlled substance and you will need to get a new prescription every 6 months if your pet is on long term therapy.
- You should not give diazepam to any other pets or household members.

Diazoxide

Proglycem® is another name for this medication.

How Is This Medication Useful?

- Diazoxide is primarily used in veterinary medicine to treat hypoglycemia (low blood sugar) caused by certain tumors (insulinomas) in ferrets.

Are There Conditions or Times When Its Use Might Cause More Harm Than Good?

- Diazoxide should not be used in patients who have low blood sugars from causes other than tumors.
- Diazoxide is similar to certain thiazide diuretics such as Lasix® and should not be used in patients that are allergic to these kinds of diuretics.
- Diazoxide should be used with caution in patients who have heart failure or kidney disease because this drug can cause changes in salt and water balance.
- Diazoxide lowers blood pressure. It should not be used at the same time as other drugs that lower blood pressure.
- Diazoxide has caused problems during pregnancy such as birth defects and delayed labor. For this reason, diazoxide should not be used during pregnancy or in nursing mothers.
- If your animal has any of the above conditions, talk to your veterinarian about the potential risks of using the medication versus the benefits that it might have.

What Side Effects Can Be Seen With Its Use?

- The most common side effects seen from diazoxide are lack of appetite, vomiting and diarrhea. These side effects can be reduced by giving the drug with food.
- Sometimes this drug can cause blood cell problems, cataracts and severe problems with water and salt balance.
- Higher doses of diazoxide can cause serious elevations in blood sugar which could be very dangerous for your pet.

How Should It Be Given?

- The successful outcome of your animal's treatment with this medication depends upon your commitment and ability to administer it exactly as the veterinarian has prescribed. Please do not skip doses or stop giving the medication. If you have difficulty giving doses consult your veterinarian or pharmacist who can offer administration techniques or change the dosage form to a type of medication that may be more acceptable to you and your animal.
- If you miss a dose of this medication you should give it as soon as you remember it, but if it is within a few hours of the regularly scheduled dose, wait and give it at the regular time. Do not double a dose as this can be toxic to your pet.
- Some other drugs can interact with this medication so tell your veterinarian about any drugs or foods that you currently give your animal. Do not give new foods or medications without first asking your veterinarian.
- **Ferrets**: Ferrets usually receive this drug orally once to twice daily.
- Other species do not typically receive this drug.

What Other Information Is Important About This Medication?

- Your pet's blood sugar level needs to be monitored while on this drug. You will need to have your pet checked every 3-4 months for adverse effects on blood cells.

Diethylstilbesterol

DES or Stilphostrol® are other names for this medication.

How Is This Medication Useful?
- Diethylstilbesterol (DES) is a female estrogen-like hormone that is used to treat urine leaking in some female dogs. It has also been used to treat certain kinds of cancer in both male and female dogs.

Are There Conditions or Times When Its Use Might Cause More Harm Than Good?
- DES and other estrogens can be very toxic to the bone marrow of dogs. Estrogens have caused the bone marrow to completely quit making blood cells and cause death in this species.
- DES can also cause a condition called pyometra which is essentially an infection of the uterus.
- Cats who have received DES for long periods of time have developed problems with liver, pancreas and heart.
- DES has caused cancer in offspring of women who took DES during pregnancy. For this reason, DES should not be used in any pregnant animal unless the benefits of treatment far outweigh the risks.
- Pregnant women should avoid all contact with DES.
- Discuss with your veterinarian about the potential risks of using the medication versus the benefits that it might have.

What Side Effects Can Be Seen With Its Use?
- DES can suppress the bone marrow causing poor production of blood cells. This may result in bruising, bleeding, anemia, and increased risk for infection.
- DES can also cause a female dog to come into "heat" and may cause some vaginal spotting. This side effect usually occurs within 1-6 weeks after starting therapy.
- If you notice any signs of tiredness, fever, vomiting, vaginal discharge, excessive water drinking or bruising and bleeding you should notify your veterinarian immediately.

How Should It Be Given?
- The successful outcome of your animal's treatment with this medication depends upon your commitment and ability to administer it exactly as the veterinarian has prescribed. Please do not skip doses or stop giving the medication. If you have difficulty giving doses consult your veterinarian or pharmacist who can offer administration techniques or change the dosage form to a type of medication that may be more acceptable to you and your animal.
- If you miss a dose of this medication you should give it as soon as you remember it, but if it is within a few hours of the regularly scheduled dose, wait and give it at the regular time. Do not double a dose as this can be toxic to your pet.
- Some other drugs can interact with this medication so tell your veterinarian about any drugs or foods that you currently give your animal. Do not give new foods or medications without first asking your veterinarian.
- **Dogs and Cats**: Dogs usually receive this medication by mouth once daily until the urine leaking has stopped and then is given only once or twice weekly as needed. Cats do not usually receive this medication as they are likely to develop heart, liver and pancreas problems as a result.
- **Horses**: Horses do not receive this medication.

What Other Information Is Important About This Medication?
- This drug is not commercially available and must be compounded by a compounding pharmacist.
- If you are pregnant or trying to become pregnant, you should not touch this medication at any time as it may cause cancer in your baby.
- DES should be stored in a tight, light resistant, child proof container away from all children and other household pets
- This drug is strictly forbidden to be used in any animal that might be used for food.

Digoxin

Lanoxin® and Cardoxin® are other names for this medication.

How Is This Medication Useful?

- In animals with congestive heart failure, Digoxin is used to help the heart beat more strongly and move blood through the body better.
- It is also used to treat certain types of heart rhythm disturbances.
- Because of its potential for toxicity and the availability of other drugs to treat heart problems in animals, this drug is being used less often now.

Are There Conditions or Times When Its Use Might Cause More Harm Than Good?

- This drug must not be given to animals who already have too much in their bloodstream. Digoxin toxicity can be fatal.
- Digoxin must not be used in animals who have ventricular fibrillation.
- Collie-breed dogs may be more sensitive to the central nervous system effects of digoxin and it should be used cautiously in those breeds.
- Many veterinary cardiologists feel that digoxin should not be used in cats with a certain type of heart disease (hypertrophic cardiomyopathy) as it may make the disease worse.
- Digoxin must be used very cautiously in animals with kidney disease, severe lung disease, and thyroid disease.
- Digoxin must be used very carefully in animals whose electrolytes (sodium, potassium, chloride, calcium) in their bloodstream are out of balance.
- While digoxin is used to treat heart failure, there are several heart conditions where it must be used very cautiously. Your veterinarian will discuss the risks of using this drug when those conditions are present.

What Side Effects Can Be Seen With Its Use?

- Most side effects of digoxin occur when there is too much drug in the bloodstream. These effects can range from mild gastrointestinal effects (lack of appetite, vomiting, diarrhea), to lethargy (lacking energy) or behavior changes to serious heart rhythm abnormalities. Because digoxin toxicity can be very serious, contact your veterinarian immediately if your animal develops any of these signs so that he for she can be sure that the medication is not becoming toxic to your animal.
- Digoxin can cause some gastrointestinal effects (lack of appetite, vomiting, diarrhea) without blood levels being too high, but contact your veterinarian to be sure.
- Cats may be more sensitive to the side effects of digoxin than are dogs.

How Should It Be Given?

- The successful outcome of your animal's treatment with this medication depends upon your commitment and ability to administer it exactly as the veterinarian has prescribed. Please do not skip doses or stop giving the medication. If you have difficulty giving doses consult your veterinarian or pharmacist who can offer administration techniques or change the dosage form to a type of medication that may be more acceptable to you and your animal.
- If you miss a dose of this medication you should give it as soon as you remember it, but if it is within a few hours of the regularly scheduled dose, wait and give it at the regular time. Do not double a dose, as this can be toxic to your pet.
- Many other drugs interact with this medication, you should tell your veterinarian about any drugs or foods that you currently give your animal. Do not give new foods or medications without first asking your veterinarian.
- It is important to monitor the amount of digoxin and electrolytes (sodium, potassium, calcium, chloride) in your animal's blood, both to maximize the drug's therapeutic benefit and to minimize the risk of toxicity. Your veterinarian will want to schedule these tests to be performed while your animal is taking digoxin
- **Dogs and Cats**: Dogs usually receive this drug orally twice daily. Cats usually receive this drug orally twice daily to once every other day.
- **Horses**: Digoxin may be used twice daily once the horse is stabilized. It is considered a Class 4 drug by the Association of Racing Commissioners International (ARCI).
- **Ferrets**: Digoxin is given orally once or twice a day to ferrets.

What Other Information Is Important About This Medication?

- The veterinary labeled digoxin elixir (Cardoxin®) is available in two separate strengths. One is three times more concentrated than the other so do not confuse the two.
- Cats generally dislike the taste of the oral elixirs.
- Digoxin products should be stored at room temperature in a tight, light resistant, childproof container away from all children and other household pets.
- If you switch between the veterinary brands and human brands, consult your veterinarian for advice on monitoring your pet during the change.

Diltiazem

Cardizem® and Dilacor® are other names for this medication.

How Is This Medication Useful?
- Diltiazem allows the heart to work more efficiently and is used to treat heart disease in dogs and cats.

Are There Conditions or Times When Its Use Might Cause More Harm Than Good?
- Diltiazem is removed from the body by the liver and kidneys and should be used cautiously in pets who have liver or kidney disease.
- If your pet already has a very low blood pressure or a condition known as "AV block", diltiazem is probably not the best drug for your pet.
- Diltiazem has caused birth defects in animals and should not be used in pregnancy.
- If your animal has any of the above conditions, talk to your veterinarian about the potential risks of using the medication versus the benefits that it might have.

What Side Effects Can Be Seen With Its Use?
- Diltiazem does not have many side effects, but the most common one is a very slow heart rate.
- Sometimes diltiazem can cause stomach upset, low blood pressure, irregular heart rate, rashes and abnormal liver tests.

How Should It Be Given?
- The successful outcome of your animal's treatment with this medication depends upon your commitment and ability to administer it exactly as the veterinarian has prescribed. Please do not skip doses or stop giving the medication. If you have difficulty giving doses consult your veterinarian or pharmacist who can offer administration techniques or change the dosage form to a type of medication that may be more acceptable to you and your animal.

- If you miss a dose of this medication you should give it as soon as you remember it, but if it is within a few hours of the regularly scheduled dose, wait and give it at the regular time. Do not double a dose as this can be toxic to your pet.
- Some other drugs can interact with this medication so tell your veterinarian about any drugs or foods that you currently give your animal. Do not give new foods or medications without first asking your veterinarian.
- **Dogs and Cats**: Dogs usually receive this medication as a "long acting form" (Dilacor®) twice daily or as the non-long-acting form three times daily. Cats may receive the long acting form as Cardizem® once daily or Dilacor® XR twice daily. Cats should receive the non-long-acting form three times daily.
- **Horses**: Horses do not receive diltiazem.

What Other Information Is Important About This Medication?
- All forms of diltiazem should be stored in a tight, light resistant, child proof container away from all children and other household pets
- Dilacor® capsules contain a given amount of long acting 'tablets" within the capsule. Your veterinarian or pharmacist will tell you how to open up the capsule and how to administer the tablets within.
- Cardizem® capsules will contain fixed proproportions of long versus immediate acting "beads" within the capsule. Your pharmacist or veterinarian will tell you how to open up the capsule and how to measure the beads for the appropriate dose for your pet.
- Long acting forms of diltiazem should not be crushed prior to administration.

Diphenhydramine

Benadryl® is another name for this medication.

How Is This Medication Useful?

- Diphenhydramine is primarily used to treat signs associated with allergic reactions to drugs or to environmental allergens.
- Diphenhydramine may be used as a treatment or preventative for motion sickness.
- It is occasionally used as a tranquilizer to calm excited animals or to treat signs (such as tremors or rigidity) associated with certain drugs or toxins.

Are There Conditions or Times When Its Use Might Cause More Harm Than Good?

- Diphenhydramine should be used with caution in patients with glaucoma as it may worsen this condition.
- Diphenhydramine should also be used with caution in animals that have problems urinating, have prostate enlargement, thyroid problems or heart disease.
- Working dogs (*e.g.,* guide dogs, search dogs, hunting dogs, sled dogs, rescue dogs) may become overly sedated and unable to perform their duties while on this drug.
- If your animal has any of the above conditions, talk to your veterinarian about the potential risks of using the medication versus the benefits that it might have.

What Side Effects Can Be Seen With Its Use?

- The most common side effect, which is desirable in many cases, is sleepiness and sedation. Most animals will become tolerant to this effect with time and the sleepiness will wear off.
- Dry mouth and inability to urinate are also a possible side effect.
- Infrequently, diphenhydramine may cause gastrointestinal distress such as vomiting, decreased appetite or diarrhea.
- Cats may become unusually excited while taking this drug.
- Animals receiving diphenhydramine will have a reduced response to allergy testing. Diphenhydramine should be stopped at least 4 days before allergy tests are started.

How Should It Be Given?

- The successful outcome of your animal's treatment with this medication depends upon your commitment and ability to administer it exactly as the veterinarian has prescribed. If you have difficulty giving any doses, please do not skip doses or stop giving the medication. Consult your veterinarian or pharmacist who can offer administration techniques or change the dosage form to a type of medication that may be more acceptable to you and your animal.
- Most cats despise the taste of diphenhydramine liquid and getting cats to accept this drug is a challenge.
- If you miss a dose of this medication you should give it as soon as you remember it, but if it is within a few hours of the regularly scheduled dose, wait and give it at the regular time. Do not double a dose as this can be toxic to your pet.
- Some other drugs can interact with this medication so tell your veterinarian about any drugs or foods that you currently give your animal. Do not give new foods or medications without first asking your veterinarian.
- **Dogs and Cats**: Dogs and cats usually receive this drug orally up to three times daily as a tablet, capsule or liquid.
- **Horses**: Horses usually only receive this drug via injection to treat an allergic reaction.

What Other Information Is Important About This Medication?

- Diphenhydramine should be stored in a tight, light resistant, childproof container away from all children and other household pets.
- Keep at room temperature, do not allow the liquid to freeze.

VETERINARY DRUG HANDBOOK-Client Information Edition
Permission to photocopy for individual clients granted by Gigi Davidson and Donald C. Plumb © 2003

Doxepin

Sinequan® is another name for this medication.

How Is This Medication Useful?

- Doxepin is a tricyclic antidepressant medication that also has some antihistamine and drying effects. It is occasionally used for treating certain skins conditions in dogs where anxiety may play a role.

Are There Conditions or Times When Its Use Might Cause More Harm Than Good?

- Doxepin should not be used in animals who have had prior sensitivity reactions to it or other drugs like it (tricyclics such as clomipramine or amitriptyline).
- It should also probably not be used in animals that have problems urinating, or that have glaucoma.
- Doxepin should not be used in animals who are also receiving drugs known as MAO inhibitors (Mitaban® Dip, Preventic® Flea Collars, Anipryl®, and isoniazid are a few of these drugs). When doxepin is given with these drugs it can cause serious increases in blood pressure that can cause death. Aged cheese can also cause this effect, so make sure that your pets do not get into any aged cheese while on this drug. If your pet is receiving any of these medications, your veterinarian will ask you to stop giving them for at least 2-5 weeks before he prescribes doxepin.
- Working dogs (e.g., guide dogs, search dogs, hunting dogs, sled dogs, rescue dogs) may become overly sedated and unable to perform their duties while on this drug.
- Doxepin's safety during pregnancy has not been proven and it probably should not be given to nursing mothers.
- If your animal has any of the above conditions, talk to your veterinarian about the potential risks of using the medication versus the benefits that it might have.

What Side Effects Can Be Seen With Its Use?

- The most common side effects in dogs include sleepiness and lethargy (lacking energy), vomiting, and hyperexcitability. Most animals will become tolerant to these effects with time and the sleepiness should wear off.
- Dry mouth and difficulty with urinating are also possible side effects.
- Contact your veterinarian if side effects are severe or persist.

How Should It Be Given?

- The successful outcome of your animal's treatment with this medication depends upon your commitment and ability to administer it exactly as the veterinarian has prescribed. If you have difficulty giving any doses, please do not skip doses or stop giving the medication. Consult your veterinarian or pharmacist who can offer administration techniques or change the dosage form to a type of medication that may be more acceptable to you and your animal.
- If you miss a dose of this medication you should give it as soon as you remember it, but if it is within a few hours of the regularly scheduled dose, wait and give it at the regular time. Do not double a dose as this can be toxic to your pet.
- Some other drugs can interact with this medication so tell your veterinarian about any drugs or foods that you currently give your animal. Do not give new foods or medications without first asking your veterinarian.
- **Dogs and Cats**: Dogs usually receive this drug orally two times daily as a liquid or capsules. Cats usually don't receive doxepin. Do not give your pet aged cheese or use tick collars while on this drug.

What Other Information Is Important About This Medication?

- Doxepin should be stored in tight, light resistant containers at room temperature.
- Doxepin can be very toxic in overdose situations. Keep out of the reach of children and other animals in the household. Store in a childproof container.

Doxycycline

Vibramycin® is another name for this medication.

How Is This Medication Useful?

- Doxycycline is used to treat many infections in pets, especially those diseases caused by ticks.
- Doxycycline can also be inserted into gum pockets of dogs after they have a dental surgery to help fight bacteria that cause periodontal disease.

Are There Conditions or Times When Its Use Might Cause More Harm Than Good?

- Some animals are allergic to doxycycline. If your animal has shown allergies to any of the tetracycline products, you should tell your veterinarian before you give your pet doxycycline.
- Because animals do not swallow their medications with water, and because their bodies are horizontal instead of vertical, tablets and capsules can sometimes get stuck on their way to the stomach. Doxycycline tablets and capsules have caused severe irritation of the throat of cats that were given these medications without water. Cats should be given about a teaspoonful of water after each tablet or capsule dose. You should offer your cat a favorite drink following each tablet or capsule dose of doxycycline. Another possibility is to always ask for doxycycline in a liquid form for your cat.
- You should always give all of the medication as directed by your veterinarian. If the entire course of treatment is not finished, the germ causing the infection may become stronger than the antibiotics and cause a worsening infection.
- If your animal has any of the above conditions, talk to your veterinarian about the potential risks of using the medication versus the benefits that it might have.

What Side Effects Can Be Seen With Its Use?

- Nausea and vomiting are the most common side effects seen with dogs and cats given doxycycline. To reduce these side effects, give each dose with a meal. If your dog or cat experiences severe vomiting or diarrhea, contact your veterinarian.

How Should It Be Given?

- The successful outcome of your animal's treatment with this medication depends upon your commitment and ability to administer it exactly as the veterinarian has prescribed. Please do not skip doses or stop giving the medication. If you have difficulty giving doses consult your veterinarian or pharmacist who can offer administration techniques or change the dosage form to a type of medication that may be more acceptable to you and your animal.
- Some other drugs can interact with this medication so tell your veterinarian about any drugs or foods that you currently give your animal. Do not give new foods or medications without first asking your veterinarian.
- **Dogs and Cats**: Dogs and cats usually receive doxycycline orally once or twice daily. Cats should be given at least a teaspoonful of water or offered a favorite liquid to drink following tablets or capsules.
- **Horses**: Horses typically do not receive doxycycline orally as it can cause some problems with the gastrointestinal tract, however it is occasionally used to treat tick-borne diseases in horses. Injectable doxycycline has caused death in many horses and should not be used until further information is available.

What Other Information Is Important About This Medication?

- Pets should be watched carefully if they spend a lot of time in direct sunlight as doxycycline can cause the skin to erupt in pustules and blisters when exposed to sunlight.

Enalapril

Enacard® and Vasotec® are other names for this medication.

How Is This Medication Useful?

- Enalapril is used to help the heart perform more efficiently by opening up the veins and decreasing fluid retention in the body.
- It is also used to protect the kidneys from certain diseases that affect the kidneys.

Are There Conditions or Times When Its Use Might Cause More Harm Than Good?

- This drug must be converted to its active form in the liver. If your pet has liver disease this drug may not be effective.
- Similarly, enalapril must be eliminated from the body by the kidneys. If your pet has serious kidney disease, your veterinarian will probably lower the dose of enalapril.
- If your pet is dehydrated, the drug may become toxic. Please ensure that your pet has lots of clean water to drink while on enalapril.
- Enalapril has caused birth defects in humans and laboratory animals. You should let your veterinarian know if your pet is pregnant or going to be bred while taking enalapril.
- Use of diuretics and other heart drugs at the same time may cause too great an effect on your pet's heart. Be sure to tell your veterinarian if your pet is on any other medications.
- If your animal has any of the above conditions, talk to your veterinarian about the potential risks of using the medication versus the benefits that it might have.

What Side Effects Can Be Seen With Its Use?

- Your pet may experience stomach upset while taking this medication.
- Enalapril may initially cause some tiredness in your pet.
- Some cats have experienced damage to the kidneys after taking enalapril.
- A dry persistent cough is a common side effect in humans but has not been reported commonly for animals. If you notice an unusual cough in your animal after starting enalapril, you should report it to your veterinarian.

How Should It Be Given?

- The successful outcome of your animal's treatment with this medication depends upon your commitment and ability to administer it exactly as the veterinarian has prescribed. Please do not skip doses or stop giving the medication. If you have difficulty giving doses consult your veterinarian or pharmacist who can offer administration techniques or change the dosage form to a type of medication that may be more acceptable to you and your animal.
- If you miss a dose of this medication you should give it as soon as you remember it, but if it is within a few hours of the regularly scheduled dose, wait and give it at the regular time. Do not double a dose, as this can be toxic to your pet.
- Some other drugs can interact with this medication so tell your veterinarian about any drugs or foods that you currently give your animal. Do not give new foods or medications without first asking your veterinarian.
- **Dogs and Cats**: Dogs usually receive this drug orally twice daily. Cats usually receive this drug orally once daily.
- **Horses**: Enalapril is not typically used in horses and is considered a Class 3 drug by the Association of Racing Commissioners International.
- **Ferrets**: Enalapril is given orally every other day to ferrets and is usually supplied in a specially compounded oral liquid to achieve the right dose.

What Other Information Is Important About This Medication?

- Enalapril should be stored in a tight, light resistant, childproof container away from all children and other household pets.
- If you switch between the veterinary brands and human brands, you should consult your veterinarian for advice on monitoring your pet during the switch.

Enrofloxacin

Baytril® is another name for this medication.

How Is This Medication Useful?

- Enrofloxacin is an antibiotic that is useful against a wide variety of infections in animals.

Are There Conditions or Times When Its Use Might Cause More Harm Than Good?

- Enrofloxacin can cause the growth plates on bones to stop growing in young animals. It should probably not be used in pets less than one year of age unless the benefits of treatment outweigh the risks of damaging growth.
- Enrofloxacin may cause damaging crystals in the kidneys of animals that are dehydrated. Dehydration may also increase the risk of seizures if your pet is taking enrofloxacin.
- Doses higher than 5mg/kg (2.2mg/lb.) per day have caused blindness in cats. For this reason, other drugs in the same class as enrofloxacin that have not yet been shown to cause blindness are generally used in cats.
- Enrofloxacin causes hallucinations in people. For this reason, if your animal suffers from any psychotic or obsessive behavior, enrofloxacin may worsen these symptoms.
- You should always give all of the medication as directed by your veterinarian. If the entire course of treatment is not finished, the germ causing the infection may become stronger than the antibiotics and cause a worsening infection. Giving enrofloxacin irregularly is very likely to cause this problem.
- Animals with decreased kidney and liver function may need to receive lower doses of enrofloxacin as these animals cannot efficiently eliminate the drug from their body.
- If your animal has any of the above conditions, talk to your veterinarian about the potential risks of using the medication versus the benefits that it might have.

What Side Effects Can Be Seen With Its Use?

- The most likely side effects seen in some animals given enrofloxacin are stomach upset, vomiting, and a lack of appetite.
- Seizures and kidney damage can occur in animals that are dehydrated.
- Dizziness and hallucinations occur in humans and may also occur in animals.

- At doses greater than 5mg/kg (2.2 mg/lb) per day, enrofloxacin can cause severe damage to cat's eyes resulting in blindness. Sometimes the cat will show dilated pupils as an early indicator of this toxicity. If you notice this in your cat, you should contact your veterinarian immediately.

How Should It Be Given?

- The successful outcome of your animal's treatment with this medication depends upon your commitment and ability to administer it exactly as the veterinarian has prescribed. Please do not skip doses or stop giving the medication. If you have difficulty giving doses consult your veterinarian or pharmacist who can offer administration techniques or change the dosage form to a type of medication that may be more acceptable to you and your animal.
- Some other drugs can interact with this medication so tell your veterinarian about any drugs or foods that you currently give your animal. Do not give new foods or medications without first asking your veterinarian.
- Any iron, aluminum, dairy or calcium products can inactivate enrofloxacin. Do not give these products 1 hour before or 2 hours after administration of enrofloxacin.
- **Dogs and Cats:** Dogs and cats usually receive this medication orally once or twice daily. Sometimes veterinarians will instruct pet owners to give injections of enrofloxacin under the skin to their pets once or twice daily.
- **Horses:** Horses may receive enrofloxacin orally once daily. Enrofloxacin, however, could potentially cause colic, and horses receiving enrofloxacin should be very closely monitored for diarrhea and signs of colic.
- **Birds:** Birds may receive enrofloxacin orally twice daily as a specially compounded liquid in a raspberry-grape or other flavored liquid.

What Other Information Is Important About This Medication?

- This drug is very bitter and may cause your pet to salivate or refuse treatment.
- Enrofloxacin should only be used in animals as it causes hallucinations in people.
- Enrofloxacin should be used very carefully in animals with a history of epilepsy.

Erythromycin

E-Mycin®, EES®, Erythrocin® and Erygel® are other names for this medication.

How Is This Medication Useful?

- Erythromycin is a macrolide antibiotic used to treat infections.
- It also stimulates movement of the stomach and bowels and is used in cases of stomach and intestinal stoppage.
- Erythromycin is also used as a topical gel to treat bacterial skin infections.
- As it inhibits certain liver enzymes that break down some other drugs, erythromycin has been used to increase the blood levels of a very expensive drug called cyclosporine so that lower doses of cyclosporine can be given.

Are There Conditions When Its Use Might Cause More Harm Than Good?

- Oral erythromycin should not be used in adult horses or in rabbits, hamsters and other pocket pets as it will kill all the helpful bacteria in the intestines resulting in fatal diarrheas.
- You should always give all of the medication as directed by your veterinarian. If the entire course of treatment is not finished, the germ causing the infection may become stronger than the antibiotics and cause a worsening infection.
- If your animal has any of the above conditions, talk to your veterinarian about the potential risks of using the medication versus the benefits that it might have.

What Side Effects Can Be Seen With Its Use?

- Erythromycin will stimulate the intestines to move and may cause cramping and diarrhea.
- It may kill off the helpful bacteria in the intestines of rabbits and hamsters and may cause a fatal diarrhea.
- It may cause a fever in foals as well as rapid breathing.
- The topical gels can cause irritation and dryness where applied. These gels should be kept away from the eyes as they are very irritating.

How Should It Be Given?

- Erythromycin should be given orally with food to decrease the likelihood of stomach upset and cramping.
- Topical gels should be used only on affected areas and kept away from eye areas.

- The successful outcome of your animal's treatment with this medication depends upon your commitment and ability to administer it exactly as the veterinarian has prescribed. If you have difficulty giving any doses, please do not skip doses or stop giving the medication. Consult your veterinarian or pharmacist who can offer administration techniques or change the dosage form to a type of medication that may be more acceptable to you and your animal.
- If you miss a dose of this medication you should give it as soon as you remember it. If it is within a few hours of the regularly scheduled dose, wait and give it at the regular time. Do not double a dose as this can be toxic to your pet.
- Because some other drugs interact with this medication, you should tell your veterinarian about any drugs or foods that you currently give your animal. Do not give new foods or medications without first asking your veterinarian.
- **Dogs and Cats**: Dogs and cats may receive erythromycin orally twice daily for infections or to lower the dose of expensive drugs such as cyclosporine. It may also be used topically as a gel on bacterial skin infections.
- **Horses**: Erythromycin is usually given orally twice daily to foals. This medication may cause a drug fever in your foal. If you notice a temperature greater than 102.7° in your foal, contact your veterinarian immediately. If you cannot reach your veterinarian, you should take measures to physically cool the foal with fans and cool water.

What Other Information Is Important About This Medication?

- Erythromycin should be stored in a tight, light resistant, childproof container away from all children and other household pets.
- Oral liquids should be shaken well and stored in the refrigerator unless otherwise instructed.

Etodolac

Etogesic® or Lodine® are other names for this medication.

How Is This Medication Useful?

- Etodolac is useful in reducing pain caused by inflammation. It is considered to be much safer than aspirin, ibuprofen or acetaminophen in dogs.

Are There Conditions or Times When Its Use Might Cause More Harm Than Good?

- Dogs with bleeding problems (e.g., Von Willebrand's Disease) should not take etodolac as it may stimulate uncontrollable bleeding.
- Animals with kidney disease should not take etodolac as it may worsen the kidney disease.
- Animals with stomach ulcers or bowel disorders should not take etodolac.
- Dogs with dry eye (keratoconjunctivitis sicca) should probably not receive etodolac as this drug may worsen the condition.
- Cats cannot efficiently eliminate etodolac and should not receive this drug as it can be toxic to the kidneys.
- Other anti-inflammatory drugs similar to etodolac have caused birth defects in humans and animals. Etodolac should probably not be used in pregnant animals.
- If your animal has any of the above conditions, talk to your veterinarian about the potential risks of using the medication versus the benefits that it might have.

What Side Effects Can Be Seen With Its Use?

- Some dogs may develop dry eye (keratoconjunctivitis sicca) after taking etodolac. If your dog develops any eye discharge or squinting while taking etodolac, you should contact your veterinarian immediately.
- Etodolac is generally free of side effects, but may cause vomiting or diarrhea in some animals. You should report these to your veterinarian immediately if they occur.
- Etodolac can cause bleeding in the gastrointestinal tract. Notify your veterinarian immediately if your pet vomits blood or has feces that appear black or tarry.
- Etodolac may cause liver damage in some animals. You should notify your veterinarian immediately if your pet seems lethargic (lacking energy), vomits, or stops eating.

How Should It Be Given?

- Etodolac should be given with food to reduce stomach injury or upset. The successful outcome of your animal's treatment with this medication depends upon your commitment and ability to administer it exactly as the veterinarian has prescribed. Please do not skip doses or stop giving the medication. If you have difficulty giving doses consult your veterinarian or pharmacist who can offer administration techniques or change the dosage form to a type of medication that may be more acceptable to you and your animal.
- If you miss a dose of this medication you should give it as soon as you remember it, but if it is within a few hours of the regularly scheduled dose, wait and give it at the regular time. Do not double a dose as this can be toxic to your pet.
- Some other drugs can interact with this medication so tell your veterinarian about any drugs or foods that you currently give your animal. Do not give new foods or medications without first asking your veterinarian.
- **Dogs and Cats**: Dogs usually receive etodolac orally once or twice daily with meals. Cats do not usually receive etodolac.
- **Horses**: Horses may receive etodolac orally once or twice daily.

What Other Information Is Important About This Medication?

- Etodolac should be stored in a tight, light resistant, childproof container away from all children and other household pets.

Famotidine

Pepcid® is another name for this medication.

How Is This Medication Useful?

- Famotidine is used to decrease acid secretion in the stomach and protect against the formation of ulcers.

Are There Conditions or Times When Its Use Might Cause More Harm Than Good?

- Famotidine should be used carefully in animals with heart disease as it may cause irregular heart beats in these animals.
- Famotidine should also be used carefully in animals with liver and kidney disease as the drug is removed from the body by these organs and may become toxic if these organs are not working properly.
- Famotidine is generally safe and effective, however it has sometimes caused damage to the red blood cells when given intravenously to cats.
- If your animal has any of the above conditions, talk to your veterinarian about the potential risks of using the medication versus the benefits that it might have.

What Side Effects Can Be Seen With Its Use?

- There are few side effects associated with famotidine but some animals may experience loss of appetite and tiredness. If your pet experiences these side effects, contact your veterinarian immediately.

How Should It Be Given?

- Famotidine should be given on an empty stomach as giving with food will cause acid secretion before the drug starts to work.
- The successful outcome of your animal's treatment with this medication depends upon your commitment and ability to administer it exactly as the veterinarian has prescribed. Please do not skip doses or stop giving the medication. If you have difficulty giving doses consult your veterinarian or pharmacist who can offer administration techniques or change the dosage form to a type of medication that may be more acceptable to you and your animal.
- If you miss a dose of this medication you should give it as soon as you remember it, but if it is within a few hours of the regularly scheduled dose, wait and give it at the regular time. Do not double a dose as this can be toxic to your pet.
- Some other drugs can interact with this medication so tell your veterinarian about any drugs or foods that you currently give your animal. Do not give new foods or medications without first asking your veterinarian.
- **Dogs and Cats**: Dogs and cats usually receive this drug orally or as an injection under the skin once daily.
- **Horses**: Horses may receive this drug as an injection once daily but generally do not receive this drug orally.

What Other Information Is Important About This Medication?

- Famotidine tablets should be stored in a tight, light resistant, childproof container away from all children and other household pets.
- Famotidine injection and oral liquids should be stored in a refrigerator.

Fenbendazole

Panacur® and Safe-Guard® are other names for this medication.

How Is This Medication Useful?

- Fenbendazole is an orally administered anthelmintic (wormer) that is effective against a variety of internal parasites in several different species.

Are There Conditions or Times When Its Use Might Cause More Harm Than Good?

- Fenbendazole should not be used in horses that will be consumed as food.
- Single doses of fenbendazole are not effective in killing the worms that infect most animals.
- Safe doses are very different for each species. Make sure that you are using the correct dose for your animal.
- Fenbendazole has been shown to promote liver tumors in laboratory rats.

What Side Effects Can Be Seen With Its Use?

- In dogs and cats, vomiting may sometimes occur after administering this medication.
- Some birds may experience bone marrow suppression after receiving fenbendazole.
- Rarely, animals may develop allergic reactions after receiving this medication especially at higher dosages. This is due to large numbers of dying parasites releasing antigens inside the treated animal.

How Should It Be Given?

- Successful treatment with this medication requires dosing for at least 3 successive days. Certain parasites may require treatment for up to 2 weeks and this drug should be given exactly as your veterinarian prescribes. Please do not skip doses or stop giving the medication or retreatment may be necessary.

- If you miss a dose of this medication you should give it as soon as you remember it, but if it is within a few hours of the regularly scheduled dose, wait and give it at the regular time; therapy will need to be extended. Do not double doses as this will not increase the effectiveness of the treatment.
- If you have difficulty administering this medication, consult your veterinarian or pharmacist who can offer administration techniques or change the dosage form to a type of medication that may be more acceptable to you and your animal.
- Some other drugs can interact with this medication so tell your veterinarian about any drugs or foods that you currently give your animal. Do not give new foods or medications without first asking your veterinarian.
- **Dogs and Cats**: Dogs and cats usually receive this drug once daily as a liquid or granules sprinkled on food. Treatment for most parasites must last for at least 3 consecutive days. Single doses do not work. Your veterinarian may ask you to also give several more days of the drug again in 3 weeks to kill the rest of the parasites.
- **Horses**: Horses usually receive this medication as an oral paste once daily for several days.

What Other Information Is Important About This Medication?

- Fenbendazole should be stored at room temperature in a tight, childproof container away from all children and other household pets.

VETERINARY DRUG HANDBOOK-Client Information Edition
Permission to photocopy for individual clients granted by Gigi Davidson and Donald C. Plumb © 2003

Fentanyl

Duragesic® is another name for this medication.

How Is This Medication Useful?

- Fentanyl is a medication that is applied as a patch that releases drug into the blood across the skin. It is used to control pain.

Are There Conditions or Times When Its Use Might Cause More Harm Than Good?

- Fentanyl should be used carefully with other drugs that cause drowsiness or depress breathing.
- Children who have peeled fentanyl patches off of pets and applied them to their own skin have suffered serious adverse reactions including death. Make sure that children and other household pets do not have access to your pet's fentanyl patch.
- Patients who have a fever may absorb more of this drug across the skin and may suffer more adverse effects. Heating pads should probably also not be used on animals with fentanyl patches as this will also increase the amount of drug absorbed.
- Fentanyl patches should not be applied on the parts where an animal will be laying down. The increased heat and pressure from laying down on the patch can increase the amount of drug released into the animal's bloodstream increasing the risk of adverse effects.
- Fentanyl is probably not safe to use in pregnancy due to the depressant effects on the fetus.
- If your animal has any of the above conditions, talk to your veterinarian about the potential risks of using the medication versus the benefits that it might have.

What Side Effects Can Be Seen With Its Use?

- Fentanyl can slow the breathing and slow the heart rate. Slowed breathing can decrease the ability of dogs to cool themselves as they cannot sweat and cool themselves by panting.
- Some animals will develop a rash at the site where the patch is applied.
- Some animals may become constipated or develop difficulty urinating.
- The effects of fentanyl on the brain may cause some animals to initially become restless or agitated, but your veterinarian can prescribe a tranquilizer to help them get through this period if necessary.

How Should It Be Given?

- The area of application will be prepared by your veterinarian by clipping. Usually your veterinarian will apply the first patch and cover it with a loose bandage. He or she will usually write the date the patch was applied on the bandage. Most patches will last cats and dogs about 3-5 days. Patches tend to last longer in cats than in dogs.
- Fentanyl patches will require at least 12 hours to take effect in dogs and 6 hours in cats. Other pain relievers should be used during this waiting period to ensure that your pet is pain-free.
- The successful outcome of your animal's treatment with this medication depends upon your commitment and ability to administer it exactly as the veterinarian has prescribed. Please do not skip doses or stop giving the medication. If you have difficulty giving doses consult your veterinarian or pharmacist who can offer administration techniques or change the dosage form to a type of medication that may be more acceptable to you and your animal.
- If you miss a dose of this medication you should give it as soon as you remember it, but if it is within a few hours of the regularly scheduled dose, wait and give it at the regular time. Do not double a dose as this can be toxic to your pet.
- Some other drugs can interact with this medication so tell your veterinarian about any drugs or foods that you currently give your animal. Do not give new foods or medications without first asking your veterinarian.
- **Dogs and Cats**: Fentanyl patches are usually placed on the animal by the veterinarian and will last 3-5 days each.
- **Horses**: Horses generally do not receive fentanyl patches outside of the clinic.

What Other Information Is Important About This Medication?

- Fentanyl patches should be stored in a tight, light resistant, childproof container away from all children and other household pets.
- You should be very careful to keep this patch out of the reach of children and humans. Application of this patch to children can result in death. If a child comes in contact with this patch, contact your physician immediately.

Fluconazole

Diflucan® is another name for this medication.

How Is This Medication Useful?

- Fluconazole is a medication that is used to treat fungal (yeast) infections of the eye and skin including ringworm.

Are There Conditions or Times When Its Use Might Cause More Harm Than Good?

- Fluconazole should not be used in patients that are allergic to it or are allergic to other antifungal agents in the same class.
- Fluconazole should not be used in patients with liver problems as it can worsen these conditions.
- Fluconazole is removed from the body by the kidneys and should be used very carefully in animals with kidney failure.
- It is probably not safe to use fluconazole in pregnancy, but you should discuss this with your veterinarian if it will save the life of a pregnant animal.
- If your animal has any of the above conditions, talk to your veterinarian about the potential risks of using the medication versus the benefits that it might have.

What Side Effects Can Be Seen With Its Use?

- Fluconazole is generally very safe when used in animals. It may sometimes cause liver problems, so your veterinarian may ask you to return to the clinic for liver function tests if your animal is taking this medication.
- Fluconazole may also rarely cause skin problems and anemias in animals. If you notice a rash on your animal or that your animal is tired or has lost interest in eating, please contact your veterinarian immediately.

How Should It Be Given?

- Fluconazole can be given with or without food and is usually given orally twice daily.
- The successful outcome of your animal's treatment with this medication depends upon your commitment and ability to administer it exactly as the veterinarian has prescribed. Please do not skip doses or stop giving the medication. If you have difficulty giving doses consult your veterinarian or pharmacist who can offer administration techniques or change the dosage form to a type of medication that may be more acceptable to you and your animal.

- If you miss a dose of this medication you should give it as soon as you remember it, but if it is within a few hours of the regularly scheduled dose, wait and give it at the regular time. Do not double a dose as this can be toxic to your pet.
- Some other drugs can interact with this medication so tell your veterinarian about any drugs or foods that you currently give your animal. Do not give new foods or medications without first asking your veterinarian.
- **Dogs and Cats**: Dogs and cats usually receive fluconazole orally twice daily with or without food. Treatment may last for weeks to months and is very expensive.
- **Horses**: Horses usually receive fluconazole orally once or twice daily while they are also receiving topical medication for eye ulcers. Therapy may last for several weeks to months and is very expensive.
- **Birds**: Birds may receive fluconazole orally once daily for weeks to months.

What Other Information Is Important About This Medication?

- Fluconazole should be stored in a tight, light resistant, childproof container away from all children and other household pets.
- Oral liquids of fluconazole should be stored in the refrigerator, shaken well and discarded after the expiration date on the container, usually 14 days.

Fludrocortisone

Florinef® is another name for this medication.

How Is This Medication Useful?
- Fludrocortisone is used to control the signs and symptoms of hypoadrenocorticism (Addison's Disease) in dogs.

Are There Conditions or Times When Its Use Might Cause More Harm Than Good?
- Fludrocortisone should not be used in pets that are allergic to it.
- Fludrocorticone may be used in pregnant mothers, however, fludrocortisone gets into the milk. Artificial milk replacer should be started after puppies have nursed colostrum.
- If your animal has any of the above conditions, talk to your veterinarian about the potential risks of using the medication versus the benefits that it might have.

What Side Effects Can Be Seen With Its Use?
- Fludrocortisone has very few adverse effects but may be irritating to the stomach. Giving with food can reduce this side effect.
- Too much fludrocortisone can cause high blood pressure and low blood potassium. If your animal seems weak or its legs appear swollen, you should contact your veterinarian immediately.

How Should It Be Given?
- The successful outcome of your animal's treatment with this medication depends upon your commitment and ability to administer it exactly as the veterinarian has prescribed. Please do not skip doses or stop giving the medication. If you have difficulty giving doses consult your veterinarian or pharmacist who can offer administration techniques or change the dosage form to a type of medication that may be more acceptable to you and your animal.
- If you miss a dose of this medication you should give it as soon as you remember it, but if it is within a few hours of the regularly scheduled dose, wait and give it at the regular time. Do not double a dose as this can be toxic to your pet.
- Some other drugs can interact with this medication so tell your veterinarian about any drugs or foods that you currently give your animal. Do not give new foods or medications without first asking your veterinarian.
- **Dogs and Cats**: Fludrocortisone is usually given orally once daily to dogs. Fludrocortisone is rarely given to cats.
- **Horses**: Fludrocortisone is rarely given to horses.

What Other Information Is Important About This Medication?
- Fludrocortisone should be stored in a tight, light resistant, childproof container away from all children and other household pets.
- Once your pet is controlled on fludrocortisone, your veterinarian may advise that you add salt to the diet to possibly lower the daily dose of fludrocortisone. Do not add salt to your pet's diet without asking your veterinarian.

Flunixin

Banamine® is another name for this medication.

How Is This Medication Useful?

- Flunixin is used to control pain and inflammation in horses and cattle.

Are There Conditions or Times When Its Use Might Cause More Harm Than Good?

- Flunixin blocks the formation of the enzymes that protect kidneys, stomach and blood cells. For this reason, flunixin should be used very carefully in animals with kidney problems, stomach ulcers and bleeding problems.
- Flunixin should also not be used in animals that are allergic to it or to other anti-inflammatory agents.
- Flunixin can be extremely toxic to dogs and cats. As there are many safer anti-inflammatory drugs available for use in these species, flunixin should probably not be used in dogs and cats.
- If your animal has any of the above conditions, talk to your veterinarian about the potential risks of using the medication versus the benefits that it might have.

What Side Effects Can Be Seen With Its Use?

- Flunixin may cause irritation and pain after injection into the muscle.
- Flunixin may cause damage to kidneys, stomach and blood cells resulting in kidney failure, ulcers and bleeding problems. The risk of these side effects occurring is increased if flunixin is used at the same time as other anti-inflammatory drugs.

How Should It Be Given?

- If given orally, flunixin should be given with food to decrease side effects on the stomach.
- If given by injection, it should not be injected into neck muscles.
- Never mix flunixin injection with other drugs in the same syringe as it may inactivate those drugs as well as itself.
- The successful outcome of your animal's treatment with this medication depends upon your commitment and ability to administer it exactly as the veterinarian has prescribed. Please do not skip doses or stop giving the medication. If you have difficulty giving doses consult your veterinarian or pharmacist who can offer administration techniques or change the dosage form to a type of medication that may be more acceptable to you and your animal.

- If you miss a dose of this medication you should give it as soon as you remember it, but if it is within a few hours of the regularly scheduled dose, wait and give it at the regular time. Do not double a dose as this can be toxic to your pet.
- Some other drugs can interact with this medication so tell your veterinarian about any drugs or foods that you currently give your animal. Do not give new foods or medications without first asking your veterinarian.
- **Dogs and Cats**: Flunixin is generally not given to dogs due to the increased risk of side effects. Flunixin should not be given to cats due to the risk of damage to the kidneys.
- **Horses**: Flunixin is usually given orally or by injection once or twice daily to horses. It should be given with food if given orally and should not be injected into the arteries due to adverse effects on the brain.
- **Cattle**: Cattle usually receive flunixin by injection once or twice daily for no more than 2-3 days. If your veterinarian uses flunixin in a meat or dairy cow, he should tell you how long to wait after the last dose before it is safe to use the milk or meat. Flunixin can cause kidney problems in humans and should be kept out of the food chain.

What Other Information Is Important About This Medication?

- Flunixin should be stored in a tight, light resistant, childproof container away from all children and other household pets.
- Flunixin injection should not be mixed with any other drugs as it may chemically inactivate itself and other drugs.
- Flunixin should not be used in beef cattle, nonlactating dairy cattle, or horses intended for food.
- Flunixin is particularly toxic to the kidneys of humans and should not be used in people.

VETERINARY DRUG HANDBOOK-Client Information Edition
Permission to photocopy for individual clients granted by Gigi Davidson and Donald C. Plumb © 2003

Fluoxetine

Prozac® is another name for this medication.

How Is This Medication Useful?

- Fluoxetine is used to treat behavior problems such as aggression and obsessive compulsive disorders in dogs, cats and birds.

Are There Conditions or Times When Its Use Might Cause More Harm Than Good?

- Fluoxetine should not be used in animals who are also receiving drugs known as MOA inhibitors (Mitaban® Dip, Preventic® Flea Collars, Anipryl®, and isoniazid are a few of these drugs). When fluoxetine is given with these drugs it can cause serious increases in blood pressure that can cause death. Aged cheese can also cause this effect, so make sure that your pets do not get into any aged cheese while on this drug. If your pet is receiving any of these medications, your veterinarian will ask you to stop giving them for at least 2-5 weeks before he prescribes fluoxetine.
- Fluoxetine can also alter the level of sugar in the blood and should be used very carefully in diabetic patients.
- Because fluoxetine is removed from the body by the liver, it should be used carefully in animals with liver disease.
- It is not known if fluoxetine can be used safely in pregnant animals. This drug gets into breast milk in high levels and should not be used in nursing mothers.
- If your animal has any of the above conditions, talk to your veterinarian about the potential risks of using the medication versus the benefits that it might have.

What Side Effects Can Be Seen With Its Use?

- Fluoxetine can cause tiredness, stomach upset, anxiety, irritability and restlessness in some animals. The most common side effect in dogs is loss of appetite. If your dog stops eating, try tempting it with better tasting foods or hand feeding until this side effect wears off. If your dog does not get his appetite back, your veterinarian will probably discontinue the use of this drug in your pet.
- Fluoxetine may cause some dogs to become aggressive. If you notice this kind of behavior change in your pet, you should notify your veterinarian immediately.

- Fluoxetine has caused liver damage in some people, so your veterinarian will probably want to monitor your pet's liver function while on this drug. If you notice that your pet seems more tired, has lost its appetite, or its skin and gums have a yellowish tint to them, you should call your veterinarian immediately.

How Should It Be Given?

- Fluoxetine can be given with or without food. Giving with food will prevent the stomach upset that is sometimes associated with this drug.
- It will take several weeks before fluoxetine reaches the blood levels required to have an effect on your pet's behavior. Your veterinarian will not be able to assess the effects of this drug for at least 1-4 weeks in your pet.
- Do not discontinue this drug abruptly. Your veterinarian will have you slowly decrease the amount you are giving over time to ensure that your pet's behavior problems do not return.
- The successful outcome of your animal's treatment with this medication depends upon your commitment and ability to administer it exactly as the veterinarian has prescribed. Please do not skip doses or stop giving the medication. If you have difficulty giving doses consult your veterinarian or pharmacist who can offer administration techniques or change the dosage form to a type of medication that may be more acceptable to you and your animal.
- If you miss a dose of this medication you should give it as soon as you remember it, but if it is within a few hours of the regularly scheduled dose, wait and give it at the regular time. Do not double a dose as this can be toxic to your pet.
- Some other drugs can interact with this medication so tell your veterinarian about any drugs or foods that you currently give your animal. Do not give new foods or medications without first asking your veterinarian.
- **Dogs and Cats**: Dogs usually receive fluoxetine orally once daily for several weeks.
- **Birds**: Birds usually receive this medication orally once daily as a liquid.

What Other Information Is Important About This Medication?

- Fluoxetine should be stored in a tight, light resistant, childproof container away from all children and other household pets.

Permission to photocopy for individual clients granted by Gigi Davidson and Donald C. Plumb © 2003

Furosemide

Lasix®, Disal® and Salix® are other names for this medication.

How Is This Medication Useful?

- Furosemide is used to remove excess fluid from the body in conditions such as heart disease, lung disease, and swelling.
- It may also be used in racehorses that get nosebleeds when they race.

Are There Conditions or Times When Its Use Might Cause More Harm Than Good?

- Furosemide should be used very carefully in animals with kidney disease as this drug may worsen the disease.
- Furosemide is related to sulfa drugs and should not be used in pets that are allergic to sulfas.
- Furosemide should be used very carefully in pets with diabetes and any other conditions where water and electrolytes are unbalanced.
- All of these conditions may be worsened if your pet is not eating or drinking enough. Please make sure that your pet has plenty of food and clean drinking water while on furosemide therapy.
- Furosemide interacts with many drugs possibly worsening your pet's condition. You should tell your veterinarian about any drugs that you are currently giving your pet.
- If your animal has any of the above conditions, talk to your veterinarian about the potential risks of using the medication.

What Side Effects Can Be Seen With Its Use?

- Furosemide may cause disruptions in electrolyte (salts) balance. Your veterinarian will monitor your animal's blood levels of potassium, calcium, magnesium and sodium.
- Furosemide can harm the nerves responsible for hearing, especially in cats. If you notice that your cat seems to have lost its balance or has a slight tilt to its head, you should notify your veterinarian immediately.
- Some animals may experience weakness from the loss of fluids and electrolytes. Other animals may experience restlessness that may be related to the increased need for urination. If your pet shows signs of excessive thirst, tiredness, restlessness, lack of urination or racing heartbeat, you should contact your veterinarian immediately.
- Rarely, animals will experience anemia from furosemide treatment.

- Dehydration may increase the likelihood of all these side effects; so make sure your pet has plenty of clean water to drink.

How Should It Be Given?

- Furosemide is usually given orally to pets that are at home. Your veterinarian will probably inject it in the clinic. Furosemide may be given orally from once to three times daily depending on the severity of disease.
- Furosemide can be given with or without food.
- The successful outcome of your animal's treatment with this medication depends upon your commitment and ability to administer it exactly as the veterinarian has prescribed. Please do not skip doses or stop giving the medication. If you have difficulty giving doses consult your veterinarian or pharmacist who can offer administration techniques or change the dosage form to a type of medication that may be more acceptable to you and your animal.
- If you miss a dose of this medication you should give it as soon as you remember it, but if it is within a few hours of the regularly scheduled dose, wait and give it at the regular time. Do not double a dose as this can be toxic to your pet.
- Some other drugs can interact with this medication so tell your veterinarian about any drugs or foods that you currently give your animal. Do not give new foods or medications without first asking your veterinarian.
- **Dogs and Cats**: Dogs and cats usually receive furosemide orally every 8-24hours.
- **Horses**: Horses usually receive this drug orally two or three times daily for fluid removal. To prevent nose bleeds, furosemide is given by injection 1-4 hours prior to a race.

What Other Information Is Important About This Medication?

- The use of furosemide in performance horses is regulated state by state. You should check with your state authorities prior to using furosemide in a performance or competition.
- Furosemide should be stored in a tight, light resistant, childproof container away from all children and other household pets.
- Furosemide is a sulfa drug and owners who are allergic to sulfas should wear gloves and exercise extreme caution while handling this medication.

Glipizide

Glucotrol® is another name for this medication.

How Is This Medication Useful?
- Glipizide is used to decrease blood sugar levels in diabetic cats. It is not effective in controlling the blood sugar of diabetic dogs.

Are There Conditions or Times When Its Use Might Cause More Harm Than Good?
- Glipizide should be used very carefully in animals with untreated diseases of the pituitary gland or adrenal gland. It is not considered effective for diabetic emergencies like diabetic coma, acidosis or ketosis.
- Glipizide has caused death to the fetuses of rats and should probably not be used in pregnant animals. It is not known if glipizide enters the milk so it should be used with extreme caution in nursing animals.
- Glipizide is not effective in treating cats that have demonstrated a resistance to insulin therapy.
- Several drugs interact with glipizide and may either increase blood sugar or excessively lower blood sugar. You should tell your veterinarian about any drugs that your cat is receiving.
- If your animal has any of the above conditions, talk to your veterinarian about the potential risks of using the medication versus the benefits that it might have.

What Side Effects Can Be Seen With Its Use?
- About 15% of cats will start vomiting when glipizide is started. This side effect usually improves after 2-5 days. If it does not improve, you should contact your veterinarian immediately.
- Initial doses of glipizide may cause your cat's blood sugar to drop too fast. If your cat shows signs of dangerously low blood sugar (hypoglycemia) such as weakness, wobbling, head tilting, shivering, sleepiness, glassy eyes, hunger or confusion, you should immediately administer 1 ml (approximately ¼ teaspoon) of Karo® syrup to the gums and get your cat to a veterinarian for emergency treatment.
- Glipizide has caused toxicity to the liver in some cats. Your veterinarian will want to monitor your cat's liver function every 1-2 weeks for a few months. It is very important that you take your cat back to the veterinarian for these life-saving rechecks. If you notice that your cat's gums or eyes have a yellowish look to them, report this immediately to your veterinarian.
- Some cats may experience bone marrow suppression from glipizide.

How Should It Be Given?
- Glipizide should be given orally twice daily with meals.
- If your cat's blood sugar values do not improve after 1-2 months on glipizide, your veterinarian will recommend that you switch your pet to insulin injections.
- The successful outcome of your animal's treatment with this medication depends upon your commitment and ability to administer it exactly as the veterinarian has prescribed. Please do not skip doses or stop giving the medication. If you have difficulty giving doses consult your veterinarian or pharmacist who can offer administration techniques or change the dosage form to a type of medication that may be more acceptable to you and your animal.
- If you miss a dose of this medication you should give it as soon as you remember it, but if it is within a few hours of the regularly scheduled dose, wait and give it at the regular time. Do not double a dose as this can be toxic to your pet.
- Glipizide is not a cure for diabetes. You will need to give this medication for the rest of the animal's life to prevent the life-threatening effects of high blood sugar.
- Some other drugs can interact with this medication so tell your veterinarian about any drugs or foods that you currently give your animal. Do not give new foods or medications without first asking your veterinarian.
- **Dogs and Cats**: Glipizide does not work in dogs. Glipizide is usually given orally twice daily to cats with meals.

What Other Information Is Important About This Medication?
- Glipizide should be stored in a tight, light resistant, childproof container away from all children and other household pets.
- Glipizide may not work forever in your cat. Many cats will stop responding to glipizide after several months and then must be treated with insulin injections.
- Glipizide is a sulfa drug and owners who are allergic to sulfas should wear gloves and exercise extreme caution while handling this medication.

Griseofulvin

Fulvicin®, Grisactin®, Grifulvin® and Gris-PEG® are other names for this medication.

How Is This Medication Useful?

- Griseofulvin is used to treat fungal conditions such as ringworm in animals.

Are There Conditions or Times When Its Use Might Cause More Harm Than Good?

- Because griseofulvin can be toxic to the liver and must be removed from the body by the liver, it should not be used in animals with liver failure or liver disease.
- Kittens are more sensitive to griseofulvin than adult cats and should be monitored very carefully while on this drug. If your kitten shows signs of weakness, loss of appetite or fever (>103°F) you should contact your veterinarian immediately.
- Cats with Feline Immunodeficiency Virus (FIV) or Feline Leukemia (FeLV) should not be treated with this drug because of an increased risk of anemia occuring.
- Griseofulvin is known to cause serious birth defects in cats. It should not be used in pregnancy as safer, more effective therapies are available.
- Griseofulvin has also been shown to decrease the sperm count and should not be used in breeding males.
- If your pet is being treated for seizures with phenobarbital, a higher dose of griseofulvin may be necessary for treatment. Please tell your veterinarian if your pet is taking any other medications.
- If your animal has any of the above conditions, talk to your veterinarian about the potential risks of using the medication versus the benefits that it might have.

What Side Effects Can Be Seen With Its Use?

- Griseofulvin can cause loss of appetite, vomiting, diarrhea, anemia, depression, weakness, incoordination and sensitivity to sunlight. If your pet is fair colored or has thin hair or shaved places, you should try to keep it out of direct sunlight for prolonged periods while on this drug.
- Griseofulvin is more likely to cause bone marrow suppression and anemia in cats than in any other species because cats lack the liver enzymes required to efficiently remove it from the body.

- Griseofulvin can cause liver damage and your veterinarian may want to monitor your pet's liver function while on this drug.

How Should It Be Given?

- Griseofulvin should be given with a fatty food to increase the absorption into the bloodstream. It is usually given orally once or twice daily for several weeks.
- Griseofulvin should be given for at least two more weeks after the symptoms have gone away to ensure that the fungus is completely eradicated.
- The successful outcome of your animal's treatment with this medication depends upon your commitment and ability to administer it exactly as the veterinarian has prescribed. Please do not skip doses or stop giving the medication. If you have difficulty giving doses consult your veterinarian or pharmacist who can offer administration techniques or change the dosage form to a type of medication that may be more acceptable to you and your animal.
- If you miss a dose of this medication you should give it as soon as you remember it, but if it is within a few hours of the regularly scheduled dose, wait and give it at the regular time. Do not double a dose as this can be toxic to your pet.
- Some other drugs can interact with this medication so tell your veterinarian about any drugs or foods that you currently give your animal. Do not give new foods or medications without first asking your veterinarian.
- **Dogs and Cats**: Griseofulvin is usually given orally once or twice daily to dogs and cats for several weeks.
- **Horses**: Horses usually receive griseofulvin orally once daily.

What Other Information Is Important About This Medication?

- Griseofulvin should be stored in a tight, light resistant, childproof container away from all children and other household pets.
- Griseofulvin comes in two different forms: microsize and ultramicrosize. The dose for each form is extremely different so you should be sure that your pet is receiving the form that your veterinarian intended, to avoid failure of therapy or toxicity.

VETERINARY DRUG HANDBOOK-Client Information Edition
Permission to photocopy for individual clients granted by Gigi Davidson and Donald C. Plumb © 2003

Hydralazine

Apresoline® is another name for this medication.

How Is This Medication Useful?

- In animals with congestive heart failure, hydralazine may be used, oftentimes along with other medications. Hydralazine works by relaxing the arteries which allows the blood to flow more easily through the body.
- Hydralazine is also used to treat systemic hypertension (high blood pressure).

Are There Conditions or Times When Its Use Might Cause More Harm Than Good?

- Hydralazine should not be used in animals allergic to it.
- It should not be used in animals whose blood pressure is already too low.
- Hydralazine should be used with caution in animals with liver or kidney disease and those who have autoimmune diseases (e.g., lupus)

What Side Effects Can Be Seen With Its Use?

- Hydralazine may cause hypotension (too low blood pressure) and then a reflex increase in heart rate. Notify your veterinarian if your animal appears weak or lethargic (lacking energy).
- If it is not given with a diuretic, hydralazine can cause sodium and water retention. Your veterinarian will probably prescribe a diuretic to be given with hydralazine.
- Hydralazine may cause decreased appetite, vomiting or diarrhea in some animals.

How Should It Be Given?

- The successful outcome of your animal's treatment with this medication depends upon your commitment and ability to administer it exactly as the veterinarian has prescribed. Please do not skip doses or stop giving the medication. If you have difficulty giving doses consult your veterinarian or pharmacist who can offer administration techniques or change the dosage form to a type of medication that may be more acceptable to you and your animal.
- If you miss a dose of this medication you should give it as soon as you remember it, but if it is within a few hours of the regularly scheduled dose, wait and give it at the regular time. Do not double a dose, as this can be toxic to your pet.
- Some other drugs can interact with this medication so tell your veterinarian about any drugs or foods that you currently give your animal. Do not give new foods or medications without first asking your veterinarian.
- Preferably give this medication with food as more of the drug is absorbed and it may reduce the chances of gastrointestinal upset occurring.
- **Dogs and Cats**: Dogs usually receive this drug orally two to three times daily. Cats usually receive this drug orally twice daily.
- **Horses**: Hydralazine is not usually used in horses.

What Other Information Is Important About This Medication?

- Hydralazine should be stored at room temperature in a tight, light resistant, childproof container away from all children and other household pets.

Hydrocodone

Hycodan® and Tussigon® are other names for this medication.

How Is This Medication Useful?

- Hydrocodone is a narcotic drug used primarily as a cough suppressant in animals with harsh, non-productive coughs such as kennel cough, collapsing trachea, and viral lung infections.

Are There Conditions or Times When Its Use Might Cause More Harm Than Good?

- Hydrocodone should not be used at the same time as drugs known as MAO inhibitors (Mita-ban® Dip, Preventic® Flea Collars, Anipryl®, and isoniazid are a few of these drugs). When hydrocodone is given with these drugs it can cause serious increases in blood pressure that can cause death. Aged cheese can also cause this effect, so make sure that your pets do not get into any aged cheese while on this drug. If your pet is receiving any of these medications, your veterinarian will ask you to stop giving them for at least 2-5 weeks before he prescribes hydrocodone.

- Because hydrocodone inibits the intestines from efficient elimination, it should not be given to animals with diarrhea caused by a toxin (poison). Once the toxin is eliminated, hydrocodone can be safely given.

- Hydrocodone and all narcotic drugs should be used carefully in animals with thyroid disease, kidney disease or Addison's disease.

- Hydrocodone can also decrease the efficiency of the lungs. It should be used with caution in animals with pneumonia or other respiratory conditions where mucous needs to be coughed out. Because dogs and cats cannot sweat and use panting to cool themselves, hydrocodone should be used with caution in dogs and cats that are exposed to hot temperatures.

- The lungs are also used to eliminate acid from the blood, and hydrocodone should be used with caution in animals with too much acid in their blood (acidosis).

- Hydrocodone and other narcotics should also be used with caution in animals that have had head injuries as the side effects from these drugs may make it difficult to assess the extent of injuries to the brain.

- Other drugs that depress the brain or lungs may increase the effects of hydrocodone on these organs. You should tell your veterinarian about any other drugs that your pet may be receiving.

- Hydrocodone may mask coughs that are used to diagnose other diseases such as heartworm disease and should not be given without a veterinarian's prescription.

- If your animal has any of the above conditions, talk to your veterinarian about the potential risks of using the medication versus the benefits that it might have.

What Side Effects Can Be Seen With Its Use?

- Typical side effects from hydrocodone include sleepiness, constipation, and stomach upset.

- While some humans have becomed addicted to narcotics while taking this drug, this has not been reported in pets.

How Should It Be Given?

- Hydrocodone should be given with food to decrease stomach upset. It is generally given no more than four times daily.

- The successful outcome of your animal's treatment with this medication depends upon your commitment and ability to administer it exactly as the veterinarian has prescribed. Please do not skip doses or stop giving the medication. If you have difficulty giving doses consult your veterinarian or pharmacist who can offer administration techniques or change the dosage form to a type of medication that may be more acceptable to you and your animal.

- If you miss a dose of this medication you should give it as soon as you remember it, but if it is within a few hours of the regularly scheduled dose, wait and give it at the regular time. Do not double a dose as this can be toxic to your pet.

- Some other drugs can interact with this medication so tell your veterinarian about any drugs or foods that you currently give your animal. Do not give new foods or medications without first asking your veterinarian.

- **Dogs and Cats**: Hydrocodone is usually given orally up to four times daily with food in dogs. It is not commonly used in cats. Do not give your pet aged cheese or use tick collars while on this drug.

- **Horses**: Hydrocodone is typically not used.

What Other Information Is Important About This Medication?

- Hydrocodone is a Class III Controlled substance and is controlled by the Drug Enforcement Administration (DEA). You will need to get a new prescription for this medication every 6 months.

- Hydrocodone should be stored in a tight, light resistant, childproof container away from all children and other household pets.

- It should not be given to anyone other than the animal for which it was prescribed.

Hydroxyzine

Atarax® and Vistaril® are other names for this medication. Atarax® is hydroxyzine hydrochloride and Vistaril® is hydroxyzine pamoate.

How Is This Medication Useful

- Hydroxyzine is an antihistamine drug used to treat animals suffering from itching and inflammation usually caused by skin disease. Atopic dermatitis is a condition for which this drug is commonly prescribed. Some salts of hydroxyzine are considerably more expensive than others, but all salts are generally considered interchangeable in animals.

Are There Conditions or Times When Its Use Might Cause More Harm Than Good?

- Because of its effect of relaxing some types of muscle, hydroxyzine should not be used in animals with enlarged prostates, bladder blockage, severe heart disease or stomach obstruction.
- Hydroxyzine has also caused birth defects in laboratory animals and should probably not be used in pregnancy. It is not known if hydroxyzine gets into milk and should be used very carefully in nursing mothers.
- As hydroxyzine causes sedation, it should be used with extreme caution in working animals such as horses and dogs.
- Hydroxyzine has caused seizures in some dogs and probably should not be used in dogs with a history of seizures.
- If your animal has any of the above conditions, talk to your veterinarian about the potential risks of using the medication versus the benefits that it might have.

What Side Effects Can Be Seen With Its Use?

- The most likely side effects are sedation and drowsiness. These side effects are generally mild and go away with time.
- Occasionally, hydroxyzine causes some animals to become overly excited. Some dogs will develop muscle tremors and seizures from this medication. Your veterinarian may want to try a test dose in your pet before long-term use, especially in horses.
- Cats have been reported to drink more water while receiving this drug and also experience behavior changes while receiving hydroxyzine.

How Should It Be Given?

- Hydroxyzine is usually given orally twice to three times daily in dogs, cats, horses and birds. It may be given with or without food.
- If your pet is a show animal or a working animal, you may want to try a test dose at home to see what effects the drug has. You may want to postpone any performances until the side effects have worn off.
- The successful outcome of your animal's treatment with this medication depends upon your commitment and ability to administer it exactly as the veterinarian has prescribed. Please do not skip doses or stop giving the medication. If you have difficulty giving doses consult your veterinarian or pharmacist who can offer administration techniques or change the dosage form to a type of medication that may be more acceptable to you and your animal.
- If you miss a dose of this medication you should give it as soon as you remember it, but if it is within a few hours of the regularly scheduled dose, wait and give it at the regular time. Do not double a dose as this can be toxic to your pet.
- Some other drugs can interact with this medication so tell your veterinarian about any drugs or foods that you currently give your animal. Do not give new foods or medications without first asking your veterinarian.
- **Dogs and Cats**: Dogs and cats usually receive this drug orally twice to three times daily.
- **Horses**: Horses usually receive this drug orally twice daily. It may be banned in some performance horses, so you should check your state or organizational guidelines prior to using in a performance or competition.

What Other Information Is Important About This Medication?

- Hydroxyzine is a Class 2 drug in the ARCI (Association of Racing Commissioners International) uniform classification guidelines.
- Hydroxyzine should be stored in a tight, light resistant, childproof container away from all children and other household pets.

Permission to photocopy for individual clients granted by Gigi Davidson and Donald C. Plumb © 2003

Imipramine

Tofranil® is another name for this medication.

How Is This Medication Useful?

- Imipramine is an antidepressant used to treat urinary leaking or separation anxiety in dogs and cats.
- It can be used to treat narcolepsy in horses.
- Imipramine is also used to treat ejaculatory problems in male breeding animals.
- It has sometimes been used in addition to other pain killers to treat cancer pain in animals.

Are There Conditions or Times When Its Use Might Cause More Harm Than Good?

- Imipramine can be very toxic in overdoses, causing heart failure and death. It should be given exactly as your veterinarian prescribes.
- Imipramine may worsen seizures in epileptic animals and should probably not be used in animals with a history of seizures.
- Imipramine should not be used in animals who are also receiving drugs known as MAO inhibitors (Mitaban® Dip, Preventic® Flea Collars, Anipryl®, and isoniazid are a few of these drugs). When imipramine is given with these drugs it can cause serious increases in blood pressure that can cause death. Aged cheese can also cause this effect, so make sure that your pets do not get into any aged cheese while on this drug. If your pet is receiving any of these medications, your veterinarian will ask you to stop giving them for at least 2-5 weeks before he prescribes imipramine.
- Because imipramine is eliminated from the body by the liver, it should be used carefully in animals with liver disease.
- Imipramine has been shown to cause bone defects in the offspring of mothers receiving imipramine during pregnancy. It should not be used in pregnancy unless the benefits to the mother outweigh the risks to the fetus. Imipramine also gets into milk at high levels and should not be given to nursing mothers.
- If your animal has any of the above conditions, talk to your veterinarian about the potential risks of using the medication versus the benefits that it might have.

What Side Effects Can Be Seen With Its Use?

- Imipramine primarily causes sedation in animals, but this side effect usually goes away with time.

- Because of its effects on certain types of tissues, it may also cause side effects such as dry mouth, urinary retention and changes in heartbeat. You should contact your veterinarian immediately if you notice any of these symptoms in your pet.
- Some animals may get diarrhea from imipramine.
- Imipramine may cause bone marrow suppression and anemia in some animals.

How Should It Be Given?

- The successful outcome of your animal's treatment with this medication depends upon your commitment and ability to administer it exactly as the veterinarian has prescribed. Please do not skip doses or stop giving the medication. If you have difficulty giving doses consult your veterinarian or pharmacist who can offer administration techniques or change the dosage form to a type of medication that may be more acceptable to you and your animal.
- If you miss a dose of this medication you should give it as soon as you remember it, but if it is within a few hours of the regularly scheduled dose, wait and give it at the regular time. Do not double a dose as this can be toxic to your pet.
- Some other drugs can interact with this medication so tell your veterinarian about any drugs or foods that you currently give your animal. Do not give new foods or medications without first asking your veterinarian.
- **Dogs and Cats**: Imipramine is usually given to dogs and cats orally once or twice daily. It can be given with or without food. Do not give your pet aged cheese or use tick collars while on this drug.
- **Horses**: Horses usually receive imipramine orally as a single dose prior to semen collection. It may also be given orally once daily for horses with narcolepsy.

What Other Information Is Important About This Medication?

- For horses, imipramine is a Class 2 drug under the ARCI (Association of Racing Commissioners International) Uniform Classification Guidelines.
- Imipramine should be stored in a tight, light resistant, childproof container away from all children and other household pets.

Insulin

Humilin®, Iletin® and Novolin® are other names for this medication. Insulin is available in different forms according to its potency and length of effect.

How Is This Medication Useful?

- Insulin is a protein (a chain of amino acids) produced by the pancreas that helps regulate blood sugar. Different kinds of insulin can be injected to control the blood sugar levels of diabetic animals.
- Because insulin drives potassium back into the blood cells, it is sometimes given to non-diabetic animals that have high potassium levels.
- Generally, the longer acting an insulin is, the less potent it is. Forms of insulin in increasing length of action are: regular, NPH, lente, PZI, and ultralente.
- Insulin is slightly different depending on its source (cattle, pigs, human). Your veterinarian will select the most appropriate insulin available for your pet.

Are There Conditions or Times When Its Use Might Cause More Harm Than Good?

- Because there are no alternatives to insulin therapy, there are no conditions where it should absolutely not be used.
- If your pet's blood sugar is less than 100mg/dl then you should not administer insulin.
- If your animal has any of the above conditions, talk to your veterinarian about the potential risks of using the medication versus the benefits that it might have.

What Side Effects Can Be Seen With Its Use?

- Hypoglycemia is the most common side effect of insulin. Hypoglycemia can be life-threatening. If your pet shows signs of weakness, wobbling, head tilting, shivering, sleepiness, glassy eyes, hunger or confusion, you should immediately administer Karo® syrup to the gums and get your pet to a veterinarian for emergency treatment. If your pet is having seizures from hypoglycemia, you should not stick Karo® syrup or your fingers into its mouth and get it to a veterinary clinic as fast as possible.

- Sometimes animals can develop a skin reaction to the insulin at the injection site. Rotating the injection site should decrease the likelihood of this adverse effect.

How Should It Be Given?

- Not only is each insulin different, but the onset, peak and duration times will be different for individual animals. There are many different types of insulin available and if a pet is not responding well to one type of insulin, there are many others to choose from. It may take a few tries before a veterinarian finds the one that is best for a particular animal.
- Ideally, animals are started on an insulin that has about a 12 hour duration. This allows the owner to administer two injections daily and not have the activity from the first dose overlap the activity of the second dose. During each of these 12-hour cycles, the insulin will have an onset, peak, and duration. All these times depend on the individual pet and on the type of insulin being used. With some pets, the insulin duration is close to 24 hours, so only one shot is given each day.
- How fast and how well insulin is absorbed into the blood depends upon where it is injected. Insulin should be injected subcutaneously (under the skin) and into the fatty layer that lies beneath the skin to obtain the best results. Injections into muscle, skin or vein may adversely affect your pet's blood sugar control.
- Always double-check the dose in the syringe before you inject your pet. Overdoses may be fatal.
- You might want to make a "guide" to double check how you filled the insulin syringe by making some ink marks at the proper dose on the syringe.

(continued on next page)

How Should It Be Given? (continued from previous page)

- When starting a new bottle of insulin, or when increasing the insulin dose, it's best to do it on a day when you can be home to observe your pet. The new bottle of insulin might be slightly stronger than the old one - especially if you used your old bottle for several months. And an increased dose requires observation for signs of hypoglycemia.

- Keep two vials of insulin in your house. You may break one, or you may run out over a holiday weekend and not be able to get a new vial right away. You may ask your pharmacist to divide your insulin refill into two separate vials.

- If you have two diabetic pets that use different types of insulin, double check to be sure you are giving each pet the correct insulin.

- The successful outcome of your animal's treatment with this medication depends upon your commitment and ability to administer it exactly as the veterinarian has prescribed. Please do not skip doses or stop giving the medication. If you have difficulty giving doses consult your veterinarian or pharmacist who can offer administration techniques or change the dosage form to a type of medication that may be more acceptable to you and your animal.

- If you miss a dose of this medication you should give it as soon as you remember it, but if it is within a few hours of the regularly scheduled dose, wait and give it at the regular time. Do not double a dose as this can be toxic to your pet.

- Some other drugs can interact with this medication so tell your veterinarian about any drugs or foods that you currently give your animal. Do not give new foods or medications without first asking your veterinarian.

- **Dogs and Cats**: Dogs and cats usually receive insulin injections twice daily just after meals.

- **Horses**: Insulin is rarely used in horses, but is given under the skin twice daily when used.

- **Birds**: Birds usually receive insulin injections once daily in the muscle.

What Other Information Is Important About This Medication?

- Always store insulin in the door of the refrigerator. Never let it be exposed to freezing or high temperatures. It is okay to leave the insulin out at room temperature just prior to injection.

- Never shake insulin. This can destroy the fragile insulin molecule as well as introduce air bubbles into the insulin which will break it down. Air bubbles also make it more difficult to measure an accurate dose in the syringe. Always roll the vial gently between the palms of the hand. This prevents the formation of bubbles and also slightly warms the insulin making it more comfortable for your pet when injected.

- Have your pet wear an identification tag that indicates it is a diabetic. You can add more information like the veterinarian's name and phone number.

- Know whom to contact in case of emergencies.

- If you take your pet out of the house, never leave home without sugar. This means when you're out on walks, going to the store, groomer, veterinarian, anywhere. Some people keep packets of honey or a small plastic bottle of corn syrup (Karo®) in their purse or in the glove box of the car. You can also purchase liquid glucose packets at the pharmacy. It's better to have a liquid sugar, but even little packets of table sugar would work. In an emergency, you don't want to spend valuable time trying to find some sugar.

- Many pets do not show any physical signs of hypoglycemia (low blood sugar). So, suspect hypoglycemia whenever your pet is not acting normally.

- Become very aware of your pet's "normal" behaviors. Knowing how your pet acts when it is healthy may help you determine when something is wrong.

Interferon

Intron® and Roferon-A® are other names for this medication.

How Is This Medication Useful?

- Interferon is used to treat certain cancers and viral diseases in dogs and cats. It has been used to control the signs and symptoms of herpes virus and feline leukemia in cats. Interferon has also been used to alleviate the symptoms of West Nile Virus infection in horses.

Are There Conditions or Times When Its Use Might Cause More Harm Than Good?

- Animals that have a history of allergy to interferon should not receive this medication.
- Although it is used to treat feline leukemia, interferon may also cause some anemias in cats and should be used cautiously in cats with severe anemias.
- If your animal has any of the above conditions, talk to your veterinarian about the potential risks of using the medication versus the benefits that it might have.

What Side Effects Can Be Seen With Its Use?

- When given orally, adverse effects to interferon are uncommon. Some adverse effects that have been reported in cats are loss of appetite, anemias, fever, allergic reactions, bone marrow suppression and muscle pain.
- When injected into humans, interferon has caused nausea, vomiting, dizziness, low blood pressure, skin rashes and a "flu-like" syndrome. It is not known if animals experience these side effects.

How Should It Be Given?

- Interferon is supplied as an oral liquid or a topical solution for the eye when used in cats. When used for feline leukemia, it is usually given for 7 days, then stopped for 7 days and then repeated. It may be supplied as an injection to be given under the skin every 2-3 days in dogs with cancer. You should always keep interferon in the refrigerator and not shake it as this will destroy this very fragile drug. The successful outcome of your animal's treatment with this medication depends upon your commitment and ability to administer it exactly as the veterinarian has prescribed.

- Please do not skip doses or stop giving the medication. If you have difficulty giving doses consult your veterinarian or pharmacist who can offer administration techniques or change the dosage form to a type of medication that may be more acceptable to you and your animal.
- If you miss a dose of this medication you should give it as soon as you remember it, but if it is within a few hours of the regularly scheduled dose, wait and give it at the regular time. Do not double a dose as this can be toxic to your pet.
- Some other drugs can interact with this medication so tell your veterinarian about any drugs or foods that you currently give your animal. Do not give new foods or medications without first asking your veterinarian.
- **Dogs and Cats**: Dogs usually receive this drug by injection 2-3 times weekly for cancer. Cats usually receive this drug orally or in the eye daily for alternating weeks of therapy followed by a drug "vacation" when treating feline leukemia or feline herpes.
- **Horses**: Horses have experimentally been treated with interferon after becoming infected with West Nile Virus. Adverse reactions in horses limit use of interferon to the veterinary clinic.

What Other Information Is Important About This Medication?

- Interferon should be stored in the refrigerator in a tight, light resistant, childproof container away from all children and other household pets.
- It should never be shaken or exposed to freezing or high temperatures.
- Solutions of interferon should be discarded after 30 days.

Itraconazole

Sporanox® is another name for this medication.

How Is This Medication Useful?

- Itraconazole is used to treat serious fungus infections in animals.

Are There Conditions or Times When Its Use Might Cause More Harm Than Good?

- Itraconazole should not be used in animals that have a history of being allergic to it or any other of the antifungal agents like it.
- Because itraconazole can cause damage to the liver, and because the liver is responsible for removing itraconazole from the body, it should not be used in patients who have severe liver disease. If your animal stops eating, becomes lethargic (lacking energy) or has yellow-ish gums or whites of its eyes, you should contact your veterinarian immediately.
- Itraconazole requires an adequate amount of stomach acid for dissolution and absorption into the blood. It should not be given on an empty stomach and must be given with food. Animals that are on antacids or that are not making enough stomach acid should not receive itraconazole orally as it will not be effective. If your pet must receive antacid medication, you should not give them until 2 hours after itraconazole has been given.
- Itraconazole has caused birth defects in laboratory animals. It should probably not be used in pregnant animals unless it will save the life of the mother. Itraconazole does get into milk in high levels and should not be given to nursing mothers.
- The positive effects of itraconazole may be stopped by some other drugs. Please tell your veterinarian about all drugs that your animal is taking.
- If your animal has any of the above conditions, talk to your veterinarian about the potential risks of using the medication versus the benefits that it might have.

What Side Effects Can Be Seen With Its Use?

- Loss of appetite is the most common side effect seen in dogs.
- Damage to the liver is also reported in about 10% of dogs taking itraconazole. This damage may be reversible if the drug is discontinued soon enough.
- About 7% of dogs will develop skin ulcers, inflammation of the veins, and swelling of the legs. Sometimes these effects will go away with lower doses, but sometimes may be severe enough that the drug must be stopped completely. Rarely, a serious condition called toxic epidermal necrolysis can occur that can be fatal.
- Cats generally suffer from loss of appetite, weight loss and vomiting following treatment with itraconazole. Liver toxicity is also possible and increases in liver function tests may indicate that the drug is causing liver problems. This usually goes away after the drug is stopped.
- There have recently been reports of dogs getting heart disease after administration of itraconazole.

How Should It Be Given?

- Itraconazole should be given with food orally once to twice daily. Giving the drug with a fatty food such as butter, milk or cheese will ensure that enough drug gets into the bloodstream. Antacids should not be given during itraconazole administration, as they will prevent absorption of the drug. The successful outcome of your animal's treatment with this medication depends upon your commitment and ability to administer it exactly as the veterinarian has prescribed. Please do not skip doses or stop giving the medication. If you have difficulty giving doses consult your veterinarian or pharmacist who can offer administration techniques or change the dosage form to a type of medication that may be more acceptable to you and your animal.
- If you miss a dose of this medication you should give it as soon as you remember it, but if it is within a few hours of the regularly scheduled dose, wait and give it at the regular time. Do not double a dose as this can be toxic to your pet.
- Some other drugs can interact with this medication so tell your veterinarian about any drugs or foods that you currently give your animal. Do not give new foods or medications without first asking your veterinarian.
- **Dogs & Cats**: Cats usually receive this drug orally once or twice daily. It should be given with food, preferably a fatty meal.
- **Horses**: Horses generally do not receive this medication due to great expense, but when used, it is given orally twice daily.

What Other Information Is Important About This Medication?

- Itraconazole should be stored in a tight, light resistant, childproof container away from all children and other household pets.

Ivermectin

Heartgard®, Eqvalan®, Zimectrin®, Ivomec®, Ultramectrin®, and Equimectrin® are other names for this medication.

How Is This Medication Useful?

- Ivermectin is an anti-parasite drug that is used to treat many different parasites in various species. It is used to treat and prevent blood (e.g., heartworm) and lung parasites, intestinal parasites and various kinds of mites including those that cause mange and ear mites.

Are There Conditions or Times When Its Use Might Cause More Harm Than Good?

- At doses higher than those used for heartworm prevention (greater that 6mcg/kg body weight monthly) ivermectin crosses into the brain of Collies and some other herding breeds where it can cause severe damage including coma and death. Even at heartworm prevention doses, the manufacturer recommends that Collies and Collie-crosses be observed for 8 hours for any adverse effects. If your Collie or Collie-cross exhibits signs of weakness, clumsiness, dilated pupils, trembling or pressing its head against the wall, you should take it to a veterinary clinic immediately.
- Ivermectin will kill many kinds of turtles and should not be used in this species.
- Ivermectin is also dangerous to some species of birds and should only be used in birds under the direct guidance of a veterinarian experienced in treating birds.
- Ivermectin in considered safe for use in pregnancy.
- Ivermectin should not be used in dairy animals.
- Ivermectin is generally very safe in cats, however, some veterinarians do not recommend using ivermectin at doses higher than heartworm prevention (24mcg/kg/month) in cats younger than one year due to the increased risk of neurological toxicity.
- If your animal has any of the above conditions, talk to your veterinarian about the potential risks of using the medication versus the benefits that it might have.

What Side Effects Can Be Seen With Its Use?

- When the parasites begin to die off in an animal treated with ivermectin, the animal can experience swelling, irritation and pain at the sites where the parasites are located. Dogs being treated with ivermectin to kill heartworm larvae (immature heartworms) can experience a shock-like reaction if there are large numbers of the larvae being killed at once.
- At higher doses any animal can experience nerve and brain toxicity. If your animal shows any signs of of weakness, clumsiness, dilated pupils, trembling or pressing its head against the wall, after being treated with ivermectin you should take it to a veterinary clinic immediately.
- Some animals may experience pain and swelling at the injection site. Limiting the injection to no more than 10ml will help reduce the likelihood of this effect.
- Topical use of ivermectin for ear mites in cats may cause pain and vomiting in a small number of cats.

How Should It Be Given?

- Ivermectin can be given orally as a tablets, chewable treats, oral liquids, oral pastes, and oral drenches. It may be given injectably and may also be administered as a topical solution for mites.
- If given for heartworm prevention, the animal should be tested for heartworm disease prior to giving the drug. It is then given once a month. If switching from the once daily heartworm medication (diethylcarbamazine) then you should begin ivermectin within 30 days of stopping the once daily medication.
- Ivermectin should only be given exactly as labeled on the container or as your veterinarian has prescribed.

(continued on next page)

Ivermectin

(continued)

How Should It Be Given? (continued from previous page)

- The successful outcome of your animal's treatment with this medication depends upon your commitment and ability to administer it exactly as the veterinarian has prescribed. Please do not skip doses or stop giving the medication. If you have difficulty giving doses consult your veterinarian or pharmacist who can offer administration techniques or change the dosage form to a type of medication that may be more acceptable to you and your animal.
- If you miss a dose of this medication you should give it as soon as you remember it, but if it is within a few hours of the regularly scheduled dose, wait and give it at the regular time. Do not double a dose as this can be toxic to your pet.
- If you overdose your pet you may see signs of staggering, vomiting, diarrhea, depression, or dilated pupils in dogs. You may see agitation, vocalization, loss of appetite, dilation of pupils, staggering, tremors, blindness, head-pressing, wall-climbing, and disorientation in cats. Most recover in 2-4 weeks with supportive care, but you should take your pet to a veterinary clinic immediately if you observe these symptoms in your dog or cat.
- If you miss more than 8 weeks in a row of ivermectin when using for heartworm prevention, you should start giving the drug as soon as you remember to. But you should have your pet tested for heartworms within 6 months as your pet may have become infected with heartworms during the time you did not give the drug.
- Some other drugs can interact with this medication so tell your veterinarian about any drugs or foods that you currently give your animal. Do not give new foods or medications without first asking your veterinarian.

- **Dogs and Cats**: Dogs and cats receive ivermectin orally once monthly for heartworm prevention, orally daily for certain types of mange and topically for ear mites as a single treatment that may be repeated several weeks later. You should read the labels supplied on your prescription of ivermectin very carefully and observe all instructions.
- **Horses**: Horses usually receive ivermectin orally as a paste or by stomach tube as a single dose to remove intestinal parasites.

What Other Information Is Important About This Medication?

- Ivermectin should be stored in a tight, light resistant, childproof container away from all children and other household pets.
- Ivermectin should be disposed of properly as it is very toxic to fish, turtles and other wildlife.

Ketoconazole

Nizoral® is another name for this medication.

How Is This Medication Useful?

- Ketoconazole is used to treat serious fungus infections in animals.
- Because it has a side effect of suppressing the adrenal glands, ketoconazole may also be used in treating Cushing's Disease in dogs.
- Ketoconazole may also slow down the elimination of certain expensive drugs (e.g., cyclosporine) from the body and may be given with these drugs to decrease the cost of long-term expensive drug therapy.
- It has also been used topically on the feet of horses with white line disease that have not responded to other therapies.

Are There Conditions or Times When Its Use Might Cause More Harm Than Good?

- Ketoconazole should not be used in animals that have a history of being allergic to it or any other of the antifungal agents like it.
- Because ketoconazole can cause damage to the liver, and because the liver is responsible for removing ketoconazole from the body, it should not be used in patients who have liver disease. If your pet stops eating, becomes lethargic (lacking energy) or looks yellow around its gums and whites of its eyes, you should contact your veterinarian immediately.
- Ketoconazole requires an adequate amount of stomach acid for dissolution and absorption into the blood. It should not be given on an empty stomach and must be given with food. Animals that are on antacids or that are not making enough stomach acid should not receive ketoconazole orally as it will not be effective. If an animal must receive these drugs, they should not be given until 2 hours after ketoconazole is given.
- Ketoconazole has caused birth defects in laboratory animals. It should probably not be used in pregnant animals unless it will save the life of the mother. Ketoconazole does get into milk in high levels and should not be given to nursing mothers.
- Ketoconazole can stop sperm production and should not be used in male animals intended for breeding.
- The effectiveness of ketoconazole may be stopped by some other drugs. Please tell your veterinarian about all drugs that your animal is taking.

- If your animal has any of the previous conditions, talk to your veterinarian about the potential risks of using the medication versus the benefits that it might have.

What Side Effects Can Be Seen With Its Use?

- Loss of appetite is the most common side effect seen in dogs and can be accompanied with stomach upset, vomiting and diarrhea.
- Damage to the liver is also reported in many dogs taking ketoconazole. This damage may be reversible if the drug is stopped soon enough.
- Some animals will experience a lightening of fur color that returns to normal when the drug is stopped.
- Ketoconazole can suppress the adrenal glands and cause symptoms of Addison's disease. Some dogs may need to have prednisone administered during treatment because of this effect.
- Cats generally suffer from loss of appetite, weight loss and vomiting following treatment with ketoconazole. Liver toxicity is also possible and increases in liver function tests may indicate that the drug is causing liver problems. This usually goes away after the drug is stopped.

How Should It Be Given?

- Ketoconazole should be given with food orally once to twice daily. Giving the drug with a fatty food such as butter, milk or cheese will ensure that enough drug gets into the bloodstream.
- Antacids should not be given during ketoconazole administration, as they will prevent absorption of the drug.
- The successful outcome of your animal's treatment with this medication depends upon your commitment and ability to administer it exactly as the veterinarian has prescribed. Please do not skip doses or stop giving the medication. If you have difficulty giving doses consult your veterinarian or pharmacist who can offer administration techniques or change the dosage form to a type of medication that may be more acceptable to you and your animal.
- If you miss a dose of this medication you should give it as soon as you remember it, but if it is within a few hours of the regularly scheduled dose, wait and give it at the regular time. Do not double a dose as this can be toxic to your pet.

(Continued on next page)

Ketoconazole

(continued)

How Should It Be Given? (continued from previous page)

- Some other drugs can interact with this medication so tell your veterinarian about any drugs or foods that you currently give your animal. Do not give new foods or medications without first asking your veterinarian.
- **Dogs and Cats**: Dogs and cats usually receive this drug orally once or twice daily. It should be given with food, preferably a fatty meal.
- **Horses**: Horses generally do not receive this medication, but when used, it is given orally once or twice daily. It may also be used topically on the feet of horses with white line disease.

What Other Information Is Important About This Medication?

- Ketoconazole should be stored in a tight, light resistant, childproof container away from all children and other household pets.
- When using the topical cream, the owner should wear gloves and wash hands after use.

Ketoprofen

Ketofen® and Orudis® are other names for this medication.

How Is This Medication Useful?
- Ketoprofen is useful in reducing pain caused by inflammation. It is considered to be safer to use in small animals than aspirin, ibuprofen or acetaminophen.

Are There Conditions or Times When Its Use Might Cause More Harm Than Good?
- Because the liver is required to remove ketoprofen from the body, this drug should be used carefully in animal's with liver disease. Your veterinarian may want to perform periodic liver function tests to show that your animal's liver is working properly.
- Dogs with bleeding problems (*e.g.,* Von Willebrand's Disease) should not take ketoprofen as it may stimulate uncontrollable bleeding.
- Animals with kidney disease should not take ketoprofen as it may worsen the kidney disease.
- Animals with stomach ulcers or bowel disorders should not take ketoprofen.
- Cats cannot efficiently eliminate ketoprofen and should not receive this drug longer than for 5 days as it will likely cause severe damage to the kidneys.
- Other anti-inflammatory drugs similar to ketoprofen have caused birth defects in animals. Ketoprofen should probably not be used in pregnant animals.
- If your animal has any of the above conditions, talk to your veterinarian about the potential risks of using the medication versus the benefits that it might have.

What Side Effects Can Be Seen With Its Use?
- Ketoprofen is generally free of side effects but may cause vomiting or diarrhea in some animals. You should report this to your veterinarian immediately if these occur.
- Ketoprofen can cause bleeding in the gastrointestinal tract. Notify your veterinarian immediately if your pet vomits blood or has feces that appear black or tarry.
- Ketoprofen is toxic to the liver in a small minority of dogs. You should notify your veterinarian immediately if your pet seems lethargic (lacking energy), vomits, or stops eating.

- Ketoprofen can be especially toxic to the kidneys of cats. If your cat vomits, stops eating, or seems lethargic (lacking energy) you should notify your veterinarian immediately.

How Should It Be Given?
- Ketoprofen should be given with food. The successful outcome of your animal's treatment with this medication depends upon your commitment and ability to administer it exactly as the veterinarian has prescribed. Please do not skip doses or stop giving the medication. If you have difficulty giving doses consult your veterinarian or pharmacist who can offer administration techniques or change the dosage form to a type of medication that may be more acceptable to you and your animal.
- If you miss a dose of this medication you should give it as soon as you remember it, but if it is within a few hours of the regularly scheduled dose, wait and give it at the regular time. Do not double a dose as this can be toxic to your pet.
- Some other drugs can interact with this medication so tell your veterinarian about any drugs or foods that you currently give your animal. Do not give new foods or medications without first asking your veterinarian.
- **Dogs and Cats**: Dogs usually receive ketoprofen orally up to twice daily for pain and inflammation. Cats do not usually receive ketoprofen for more than 5 days as they have a difficult time eliminating it from their bodies.
- **Horses**: Horses usually receive ketoprofen as a single dose.
- **Rabbits/Ferrets**: Rabbits and ferrets may receive ketoprofen once or twice daily for pain. These pets require small doses that will have to be compounded by your pharmacist.

What Other Information Is Important About This Medication?
- Ketoprofen should be stored in a tight, light resistant, childproof container away from all children and other household pets.

Lactulose

Chronulac® and Cephulac® are other names for this medication.

How Is This Medication Useful?

- Lactulose is a medication that is used as a stool softener to treat constipation. Some cats with a condition called megacolon (flaccid intestines causing constipation) may need to receive lactulose for most of their lives.
- It can also be used in liver disease to help reduce ammonia that can build up in the blood.

Are There Conditions or Times When Its Use Might Cause More Harm Than Good?

- Lactulose is comprised of sugars and may cause problems in diabetic animals. You may need to alter your pet's insulin dose when administering lactulose.
- As lactulose can cause diarrhea, it should be used very carefully in animals with fluid and electrolyte imbalances. If your pet shows signs of weakness, incoordination or irregular heartbeat, you should contact your veterinarian immediately. If your animal has any of the above conditions, talk to your veterinarian about the potential risks of using the medication versus the benefits that it might have.

What Side Effects Can Be Seen With Its Use?

- Diarrhea is the most common side effect of lactulose. You should make sure your animal has plenty of clean water to drink while being treated with lactulose to prevent dehydration.
- Some animals will become gassy and experience stomach cramping.
- Cats dislike the taste of lactulose and it may be difficult to get them to accept this medication.

How Should It Be Given?

- Lactulose is usually given orally up to three times daily. It is a sticky, sweet oral liquid that may be difficult to get into cats. To treat constipation, it should be given until the pet produces 2-3 very soft stools daily. It can also be given as an enema for patients that are in a severe liver failure crisis.

- The successful outcome of your animal's treatment with this medication depends upon your commitment and ability to administer it exactly as the veterinarian has prescribed. Please do not skip doses or stop giving the medication. If you have difficulty giving doses consult your veterinarian or pharmacist who can offer administration techniques or change the dosage form to a type of medication that may be more acceptable to you and your animal.
- If you miss a dose of this medication you should give it as soon as you remember it, but if it is within a few hours of the regularly scheduled dose, wait and give it at the regular time. Do not double a dose as this can be toxic to your pet.
- Some other drugs can interact with this medication so tell your veterinarian about any drugs or foods that you currently give your animal. Do not give new foods or medications without first asking your veterinarian.
- **Dogs and Cats**: Dogs and cats usually receive lactulose orally 2-4 times daily. Your veterinarian may also administer lactulose as an enema in the veterinary clinic, but this is generally not recommended to be performed at home.
- **Horses**: Horses may receive lactulose for liver failure and receive the drug orally up to three times daily.

What Other Information Is Important About This Medication?

- Lactulose should be stored in a tight, light resistant, childproof container away from all children and other household pets.
- Refrigeration is not required and may make the drug too thick to remove from the medication container.

VETERINARY DRUG HANDBOOK-Client Information Edition
Permission to photocopy for individual clients granted by Gigi Davidson and Donald C. Plumb © 2003

Levothyroxine

Soloxine®, Thyro-Tabs®, Thyro-L®, Thyro-Form®, and Synthroid® or L-thyroxine are other names for this medication.

How Is This Medication Useful?

- Levothyroxine is used to treat pets that don't make enough thyroid hormone.
- It has also been used to reduce weight in obese birds not responding to other therapies.

Are There Conditions or Times When Its Use Might Cause More Harm Than Good?

- Levothyroxine should not be given to animals with heart conditions or those who are producing too much thyroid hormone. It should be used carefully in animals with diabetes, Addison's disease, heart disease or in old and debilitated animals. If your pet is diabetic, you may have to adjust the amount of insulin you give after levothyroxine is started.
- If your animal has any of the above conditions, talk to your veterinarian about the potential risks of using the medication versus the benefits that it might have.

What Side Effects Can Be Seen With Its Use?

- If administered at the correct dose, levothyroxine should not cause any side effects. If too much levothyroxine is given, your pet may experience racing heartbeat, excessive thirst and urination, excessive hunger, excitation and restlessness, panting and nervousness. If your pet shows these signs, you should contact your veterinarian immediately.
- Some species of red-feathered birds may start growing yellow feathers after treatment with levothyroxine.
- Levothyroxine can severely alter the results of laboratory tests. You should tell your veterinarian that your pet is taking levothyroxine before any laboratory testing is performed.

How Should It Be Given?

- The successful outcome of your animal's treatment with this medication depends upon your commitment and ability to administer it exactly as the veterinarian has prescribed. Please do not skip doses or stop giving the medication. If you have difficulty giving doses consult your veterinarian or pharmacist who can offer administration techniques or change the dosage form to a type of medication that may be more acceptable to you and your animal.
- If you miss a dose of this medication you should give it as soon as you remember it, but if it is within a few hours of the regularly scheduled dose, wait and give it at the regular time. Do not double a dose as this can be toxic to your pet.
- Some other drugs can interact with this medication so tell your veterinarian about any drugs or foods that you currently give your animal. Do not give new foods or medications without first asking your veterinarian.
- **Dogs and Cats**: Dogs usually receive levothyroxine orally once or twice daily. Cats do not usually receive levothyroxine but may receive it for short periods of time to correct overtreatment of hyperthyroidism.
- **Horses**: Horses receive levothyroxine powder in the feed or mixed with corn syrup orally once daily.
- **Birds**: Birds receive levothyroxine in their drinking water as a 0.1mg tablet dissolved in 1-4oz of drinking water daily. Feather color may change to yellow after treatment.

What Other Information Is Important About This Medication?

- Levothyroxine should be stored in a tight, light resistant, childproof container away from all children and other household pets.

Lincomycin

Lincocin® is another name for this medication.

How Is This Medication Useful?

- Lincomycin is a type of antibiotic that is used to treat certain types of bacterial infections in dogs, cats, swine and ferrets.

Are There Conditions or Times When Its Use Might Cause More Harm Than Good?

- Lincomycin should not be used in horses, ruminants (cattle, sheep, goats), rabbits, hamsters, or guinea pigs as it may cause severe diarrhea that can cause death.
- Lincomycin should not be given to animals allergic to it or drugs like it (*e.g.*, clindamycin).
- It is not known if lincomycin is safe to use during pregnancy.
- It should be used cautiously in nursing animals as lincomycin can enter into milk and can cause diarrhea in offspring.
- You should always give all of the medication as directed by your veterinarian. If the entire course of treatment is not finished, the germ causing the infection may become stronger than the antibiotics and cause a worsening infection.
- If your animal has any of the above conditions, talk to your veterinarian about the potential risks of using the medication versus the benefits that it might have.

What Side Effects Can Be Seen With Its Use?

- The most common side effects seen in dogs or cats with orally administered lincomycin are vomiting and loose stools.
- If diarrhea becomes bloody, severe, or lasts for several days contact your veterinarian.
- Allergic reactions are possible, but very rare.

How Should It Be Given?

- The successful outcome of your animal's treatment with this medication depends upon your commitment and ability to administer it exactly as the veterinarian has prescribed. Give this drug for the full course of treatment prescribed by your veterinarian, even if your pet is better or seems cured as bacteria may remain that could make the infection worse.
- Please do not skip doses or stop giving the medication. If you have difficulty giving doses consult your veterinarian or pharmacist who can offer administration techniques or change the dosage form to a type of medication that may be more acceptable to you and your animal.

- If you miss a dose of this medication you should give it as soon as you remember it, but if it is within a few hours of the regularly scheduled dose, wait and give it at the regular time. Do not double a dose as this can be toxic to your pet.
- Because some other drugs interact with this medication, especially kaolin containing antidiarrhea medications, you should tell your veterinarian about any drugs or foods that you currently give your animal. Do not give new foods or medications without first asking your veterinarian.
- **Dogs and Cats**: Dogs and cats usually receive this drug orally two to three times daily as a tablet or liquid. Your veterinarian my also inject this medication.
- **Horses**: Horses should generally not receive this medication as it can cause severe diarrhea.
- **Rabbits, Hamsters, Guinea pigs, Gerbils**: These animals should not receive this medication as it can cause severe diarrhea and death.

What Other Information Is Important About This Medication?

- Lincomycin should be stored in a tight, light resistant, childproof container away from all children and other household pets.
- This medication may be stored at room temperature.
- It often takes a few days for this medication to reduce the signs of infection in your animal, but if your animal does not show some improvement after several days of treatment, or if their condition gets worse, contact your veterinarian.

Liothyronine

Cytomel® is another name for this medication.

How Is This Medication Useful?
- Liothyronine is used to diagnose cats with overactive thyroids. It may also be used to treat animals with underactive thyroids that do not respond to levothyroxine.

Are There Conditions or Times When Its Use Might Cause More Harm Than Good?
- Liothyronine should not be given to animals with heart conditions or those who are producing too much thyroid hormone. It should be used carefully in animals with diabetes, Addison's disease, heart disease or in old and debilitated animals. If your pet is diabetic, you may have to adjust the amount of insulin you give after liothyronine is started.
- If your animal has any of the above conditions, talk to your veterinarian about the potential risks of using the medication versus the benefits that it might have.

What Side Effects Can Be Seen With Its Use?
- If administered at the correct dose, liothyronine should not cause any side effects. If too much liothyronine is given, your pet may experience racing heartbeat, excessive thirst and urination, excessive hunger, excitation and restlessness, panting and nervousness. If your pet shows these signs, you should contact your veterinarian immediately.
- Liothyronine can severely alter the results of laboratory tests. You should tell your veterinarian that your pet is taking liothyronine before any laboratory testing is performed.

How Should It Be Given?
- Liothyronine should be given exactly as your veterinarian has prescribed. If your veterinarian has prescribed liothyronine for your cat to do a T3 suppression test, you will give the drug every 8 hours for 7 treatments and then take the cat back to the veterinarian to have a blood sample drawn within 2-4 hours of the last dose.

- The successful outcome of your animal's treatment with this medication depends upon your commitment and ability to administer it exactly as the veterinarian has prescribed. Please do not skip doses or stop giving the medication. If you have difficulty giving doses consult your veterinarian or pharmacist who can offer administration techniques or change the dosage form to a type of medication that may be more acceptable to you and your animal.
- If you miss a dose of this medication you should give it as soon as you remember it, but if it is within a few hours of the regularly scheduled dose, wait and give it at the regular time. Do not double a dose as this can be toxic to your pet.
- Some other drugs can interact with this medication so tell your veterinarian about any drugs or foods that you currently give your animal. Do not give new foods or medications without first asking your veterinarian.
- **Dogs and Cats**: Dogs do not generally receive this drug, but if so they receive it orally three times daily. Cats will receive this drug to perform a test to diagnose hyperthyroidism. You will be instructed to give your cat a dose of liothyronine every 8 hours for 7 doses. A blood sample must then be taken 2-4 hours after the last dose to determine if your cat is hyperthyroid or not.

What Other Information Is Important About This Medication?
- Liothyronine should be stored in a tight, light resistant, childproof container away from all children and other household pets.

Lufenuron

Program® is another name for this medication.

How Is This Medication Useful?

- Lufenuron stops the formation of a substance called chitin. Chitin is an important part of flea and fungus shells. Disrupting chitin will help prevent the growth of fleas and certain types of fungi.

Are There Conditions or Times When Its Use Might Cause More Harm Than Good?

- Lufenuron appears to be safe to use in dogs and cats.

What Side Effects Can Be Seen With Its Use?

- No confirmed side effects have been reported.
- There are anecdotal reports (not confirmed) of cats developing a cancerous lump at the injection site when injectable lufenuron is given.

How Should It Be Given?

- Lufenuron should be given orally once every month. It should be given with a fatty meal to ensure that it is completely absorbed into the bloodstream. It may also be given by injection to cats, although this route is controversial as it may be associated with cancer formation. If it is used to treat ringworm or other fungus infections, it should be given at a higher dose once weekly for 2-3 weeks.
- The successful outcome of your animal's treatment with this medication depends upon your commitment and ability to administer it exactly as the veterinarian has prescribed. Please do not skip doses or stop giving the medication. If you have difficulty giving doses consult your veterinarian or pharmacist who can offer administration techniques or change the dosage form to a type of medication that may be more acceptable to you and your animal.

- If you miss a dose of this medication you should give it as soon as you remember it, but if it is within a few hours of the regularly scheduled dose, wait and give it at the regular time. Do not double a dose as this can be toxic to your pet.
- Some other drugs can interact with this medication so tell your veterinarian about any drugs or foods that you currently give your animal. Do not give new foods or medications without first asking your veterinarian.
- **Dogs and Cats**: Dogs and cats usually receive lufenuron orally once monthly for flea prevention. Cats may receive lufenuron orally once weekly to help treat ringworm.
- **Horses**: Although uncommon, lufenuron may be given to horses orally or topically to assist in eradication of fungal infections.

What Other Information Is Important About This Medication?

- Lufenuron should be stored in a tight, light resistant, childproof container away from all children and other household pets.

Marbofloxacin

Zeniquin® is another name for this medication.

How Is This Medication Useful?

- Marbofloxacin is a quinolone antibiotic used to treat infections in animals.

Are There Conditions or Times When Its Use Might Cause More Harm Than Good?

- Animals allergic to marbofloxacin or drugs like it should not receive marbofloxacin.
- Marbofloxacin and drugs like it should not be used in animals that are still growing because it may affect joints and bone growth. Some infections are serious enough, however, that you and your veterinarian may wish to risk this effect.
- In high doses, marbofloxacin and drugs like it can cause blindness in cats. Your veterinarian will prescribe marbofloxacin at a safe dose, but if your cat shows any signs of dilated pupils or any change in behavior, you should contact your veterinarian immediately.
- Marbofloxacin and other quinolones may rarely cause a seizure in animals that are prone to seizures. If your pet has ever had a seizure, you should tell your veterinarian before administering marbofloxacin.
- Marbofloxacin is forbidden to be used in any animal that will be used as food for humans.
- You should always give all of the medication as directed by your veterinarian. If the entire course of treatment is not finished, the germ causing the infection may become stronger than the antibiotics and cause a worsening infection.
- If your animal has any of the above conditions, talk to your veterinarian about the potential risks of using the medication versus the benefits that it might have.

What Side Effects Can Be Seen With Its Use?

- Except for the effects mentioned above, marbofloxacin is generally free of any side effects. Some animals will suffer from loss of appetite, vomiting, diarrhea and tiredness.
- Rarely, some animals will develop liver problems after taking marbofloxacin.

How Should It Be Given?

- Marbofloxacin should be given orally on an empty stomach. Iron, antacids and dairy products should not be given within 2 hours after giving marbofloxacin.
- The successful outcome of your animal's treatment with this medication depends upon your commitment and ability to administer it exactly as the veterinarian has prescribed. Do not stop giving the antibiotics just because your pet looks better. Please do not skip doses or stop giving the medication. If you have difficulty giving doses consult your veterinarian or pharmacist who can offer administration techniques or change the dosage form to a type of medication that may be more acceptable to you and your animal.
- If you miss a dose of this medication you should give it as soon as you remember it, but if it is within a few hours of the regularly scheduled dose, wait and give it at the regular time. Do not double a dose as this can be toxic to your pet.
- Some other drugs can interact with this medication so tell your veterinarian about any drugs or foods that you currently give your animal. Do not give new foods or medications without first asking your veterinarian.
- **Dogs and Cats**: Dogs and cats usually receive marbofloxacin orally once to twice daily for several days.
- **Horses**: Horses generally do not receive marbofloxacin but may receive it orally once daily mixed with feed.

What Other Information Is Important About This Medication?

- Marbofloxacin should be stored in a tight, light resistant, childproof container away from all children and other household pets.

Meloxicam

Mobic® and Metacam® are other names for this medication.

How Is This Medication Useful?

- Meloxicam is a non-steroidal anti-inflammatory drug that is used to stop pain and inflammation in animals. Meloxicam and drugs like it have fewer side effects in animals than drugs like aspirin, acetaminophen, ibuprofen and naproxen.

Are There Conditions or Times When Its Use Might Cause More Harm Than Good?

- Animals allergic to meloxicam or drugs like it should not take this drug.
- Because meloxicam may cause stomach ulcers and bleeding, it should not be given to animals who already have stomach or bleeding problems.
- Meloxicam can also cause damage to the liver and kidneys and should be used very carefully, if at all, in animals who already have problems with these organs.
- Meloxicam should not be used in animals who are dehydrated or have fluid imbalance because this will increase the risk of damage to the kidneys.
- Meloxicam should not be used in combination with other anti-inflammatory drugs as this can increase the risk of serious side effects. Ask your veterinarian before you give any other medications to your pet while taking meloxicam.
- Meloxicam should not be used in pregnant or nursing animals unless the life of the mother is at risk. Meloxicam should not be used in animals less than 6 weeks old.
- If your animal has any of the above conditions, talk to your veterinarian about the potential risks of using the medication versus the benefits that it might have.

What Side Effects Can Be Seen With Its Use?

- Meloxicam can sometimes cause stomach upset in animals. If your pet vomits blood or appears to have blood in its stools, you should stop giving the drug and call your veterinarian immediately.

- It can also cause damage to the liver and kidneys and blood system. If your pet loses its appetite, becomes unusually tired or has changes in urination, you should contact your veterinarian immediately. If your pet shows signs of bruising on its gums and hairless areas, you should contact your veterinarian immediately.

How Should It Be Given?

- Meloxicam should be given with food.
- The successful outcome of your animal's treatment with this medication depends upon your commitment and ability to administer it exactly as the veterinarian has prescribed. Please do not skip doses or stop giving the medication. If you have difficulty giving doses consult your veterinarian or pharmacist who can offer administration techniques or change the dosage form to a type of medication that may be more acceptable to you and your animal.
- If you miss a dose of this medication you should give it as soon as you remember it, but if it is within a few hours of the regularly scheduled dose, wait and give it at the regular time. Do not double a dose as this can be toxic to your pet.
- Some other drugs can interact with this medication so tell your veterinarian about any drugs or foods that you currently give your animal. Do not give new foods or medications without first asking your veterinarian.
- **Dogs and Cats**: Dogs and cats usually receive this drug orally once daily.
- **Horses**: Horses usually receive this drug either by injection or orally.

What Other Information Is Important About This Medication?

- Meloxicam should be stored in a tight, light resistant, childproof container away from all children and other household pets. If your pharmacist has compounded a special liquid form of meloxicam, you should shake it well and store it exactly as the pharmacist has instructed.

VETERINARY DRUG HANDBOOK-Client Information Edition
Permission to photocopy for individual clients granted by Gigi Davidson and Donald C. Plumb © 2003

Methimazole

Tapazole® is another name for this medication.

How Is This Medication Useful?

- Methimazole is a medication given to cats to lower the amount of thyroid hormone. It does not cure an overactive thyroid but will control this disease if given to the animal for the rest of its life.
- It may sometimes also be given to dogs that are receiving cisplatin chemotherapy to protect the kidneys.

Are There Conditions or Times When Its Use Might Cause More Harm Than Good?

- Methimazole should not be used in animals that have shown an allergy to it or drugs like it.
- Methimazole may cause serious effects on the liver as well as the blood and immune systems. This drug should probably not be used in animals that already have anemia, liver disease, or problems with their immune system.
- Methimazole may be used in pregnant animals but may cause low thyroid function in the babies. Kittens born to mothers taking methimazole should be placed on a milk replacer after they have nursed colostrum from the mother.
- If your animal has any of the above conditions, talk to your veterinarian about the potential risks of using the medication versus the benefits that it might have.

What Side Effects Can Be Seen With Its Use?

- Most side effects happen in the first year of therapy. The most common side effect is vomiting and loss of appetite.
- Some cats will develop a skin condition from methimazole and will scratch until open bloody sores result. If you notice the development of sores on your cat, you should call your veterinarian immediately. Methimazole treatment should be stopped in these cats.
- Some animals will develop an anemia from methimazole. If you notice that your cat is unusually tired, has a fever (>103°F) or shows signs of bruising, you should contact your veterinarian immediately.
- Very rarely some cats receiving methimazole will develop myasthenia gravis, a disease that severely weakens the muscles.

How Should It Be Given?

- Methimazole is usually given orally once to three times daily as a tablet or an oral liquid. It is also frequently given as a topical gel (transdermal) that you rub into your cat's ear twice daily. If you are using the gel form of methimazole, you should always wear gloves and wash your hands well after use.
- The successful outcome of your animal's treatment with this medication depends upon your commitment and ability to administer it exactly as the veterinarian has prescribed. Please do not skip doses or stop giving the medication. If you have difficulty giving doses consult your veterinarian or pharmacist who can offer administration techniques or change the dosage form to a type of medication that may be more acceptable to you and your animal.
- If you miss a dose of this medication you should give it as soon as you remember it, but if it is within a few hours of the regularly scheduled dose, wait and give it at the regular time. Do not double a dose as this can be toxic to your pet.
- Some other drugs can interact with this medication so tell your veterinarian about any drugs or foods that you currently give your animal. Do not give new foods or medications without first asking your veterinarian.
- **Dogs and Cats**: Cats receive methimazole orally or as a topical gel once to three times daily for the rest of their life. Dogs do not usually receive methimazole, but your veterinarian may give methimazole just prior to chemotherapy to protect the kidneys.

What Other Information Is Important About This Medication?

- Methimazole should be stored in a tight, light resistant, childproof container away from all children and other household pets.
- If you are administering methimazole transdermal gel, you should wear gloves and wash hands after handling. Owners who have low thyroid function should be very careful when handling this drug and should avoid all skin contact with the drug.

Methocarbamol

Robaxin® is another name for this medication.

How Is This Medication Useful?

- Methocarbamol is a muscle relaxant used to treat muscle spasms in animals.

Are There Conditions or Times When Its Use Might Cause More Harm Than Good?

- Methocarbamol should not be used in animals that have shown an allergy to it or drugs like it (*e.g.*, Robitussin®).
- It is not known if methocarbamol can be used safely in pregnant animals.
- One of the ingredients in methocarbamol injection (PEG 300) can be very toxic to the kidneys. For this reason, methocarbamol injection should not be used in animals with kidney disease. The oral forms of methocarbamol do not have this ingredient in them and do not cause damage to the kidneys.
- Methocarbamol can cause extreme drowsiness and should be used very carefully in working animals. You should see how this drug affects your dog or horse before using the animal for work or in a performance.
- Methocarbamol can cause severe drowsiness when used with other drugs that also cause this side effect. You should not give your pet any other drugs without first asking your veterinarian.
- If your animal has any of the above conditions, talk to your veterinarian about the potential risks of using the medication versus the benefits that it might have.

What Side Effects Can Be Seen With Its Use?

- The most common side effect of methocarbamol is drowsiness.
- Other side effects include drooling, tiredness, stumbling and incoordination, and vomiting.

How Should It Be Given?

- Methocarbamol is usually given orally, but may be injected by your veterinarian at the clinic.
- The successful outcome of your animal's treatment with this medication depends upon your commitment and ability to administer it exactly as the veterinarian has prescribed. Please do not skip doses or stop giving the medication. If you have difficulty giving doses consult your veterinarian or pharmacist who can offer administration techniques or change the dosage form to a type of medication that may be more acceptable to you and your animal.
- If you miss a dose of this medication you should give it as soon as you remember it, but if it is within a few hours of the regularly scheduled dose, wait and give it at the regular time. Do not double a dose as this can be toxic to your pet.
- Some other drugs can interact with this medication so tell your veterinarian about any drugs or foods that you currently give your animal. Do not give new foods or medications without first asking your veterinarian.
- **Dogs and Cats**: Dogs and cats usually receive methocarbamol orally two to three times daily.
- **Horses**: Horses usually receive methocarbamol as an injection by the veterinarian but may also receive the medication orally. It is a Class 4 drug as classified by the Association of Racing Commissioners Interrnational.

What Other Information Is Important About This Medication?

- Methocarbamol should be stored in a tight, light resistant, childproof container away from all children and other household pets.

VETERINARY DRUG HANDBOOK-Client Information Edition
Permission to photocopy for individual clients granted by Gigi Davidson and Donald C. Plumb © 2003

Methylprednisolone

Medrol®, Solu-Medrol®, Depo-Medrol®, and Methapred® are other names for this medication.

How Is This Medication Useful?

- Methylprednisolone is a glucocorticoid drug (like the hormone cortisol) used for many conditions. Glucocorticocoids affect nearly every cell in the body and can be used to suppress the immune system in diseases like lupus, to stop itching, to treat Addison's Disease, to treat certain types of cancer, to stop swelling of the brain, to treat certain kinds of anemia and many other diseases and conditions. You should ask your veterinarian specifically why this medication is being used in your pet.

Are There Conditions or Times When Its Use Might Cause More Harm Than Good?

- Methylprednisolone and drugs like it should not be used in patients that have a fungus infection, as this will cause significant worsening of the fungal condition.
- Some kinds of mange are worsened with the use of methylprednisolone and drugs like it.
- Methylprednisolone and drugs like it should always be given with food to prevent stomach ulcers and bleeding that are sometimes associated with oral corticosteroid therapy.
- Animals with Cushing's disease are already making too much cortisol and should only receive glucocorticoid drugs during stressful events or when your veterinarian recommends them.
- Methylprednisolone and other glucocorticoids may stunt the growth of developing animals and should be used with extreme caution in young animals.
- The injectable forms of methyprednisolone should not be injected into the muscle in animals with too few platelets.
- The injectable forms should not be injected into infected joints or into other infected areas.
- Methylprednisolone and drugs like it significantly alter the effect of other medications. You should not give it at the same time as other antiflammatory drugs (NSAIDs) such as aspirin or carprofen (Rimadyl®), etodolac (Etogesic®) or deracoxib (Deramaxx®). You should always tell you veterinarian about any other medications that you are giving your pet.
- Glucocorticoids also affect the results of many laboratory tests. You should always tell your veterinarian about any medications that you are giving your pet prior to a laboratory test of any kind.

- If your animal has been on high doses of methylprednisolone or other immunosuppressive drugs, you should not have it vaccinated without your veterinarian's advice as the vaccine may not work or may actually give your pet the disease that you are trying to prevent.
- Animals who have received methylprednisolone or drugs like it for a long time should not be taken off the drug suddenly as their bodies may not return to making their own cortisol hormone. Cortisol or methylprednisolone help your animal handle stressful events so you should ask your veterinarian before stopping any methylprednisolone therapy.
- Methylprednisolone and drugs like it should be used very carefully in diabetic pets as these drugs will alter blood sugar and the amount of insulin that your pet needs.
- Methylprednisolone therapy may cause your horse to go into early labor if administered during the later parts of pregnancy.
- If your animal has any of the above conditions, talk to your veterinarian about the potential risks of using the medication versus the benefits that it might have.

What Side Effects Can Be Seen With Its Use?

- Animals treated with methylprednisolone will have an increased appetite, increased thirst and an increased need to urinate. You should be aware that your pet may need to go out more frequently to urinate. As it is stressful to some pets to have "accidents" you should make sure that your pet can go outside or have a clean litter box when needed.
- Glucocorticoid drugs will suppress your animal's immune system and may increase the risk for infection. If your pet shows any signs of fever (103-105°F in most dogs and cats), or acts like it has a urinary tract infection (frequent or painful urination) you should contact your veterinarian immediately.

(Continued on following page)

Methylprednisolone
(continued)

What Side Effects Can Be Seen With Its Use? (continued from previous page)

- Some animals on long-term therapy with methylprednisolone will develop Cushing's disease. If your pet shows signs of dry hair coat or hair loss, weakness and muscle loss, darkening of the skin, or develops a pot-belly, you should contact your veterinarian.
- Some animals may become aggressive while on methylprednisolone. You should contact your veterinarian if this behavior change occurs or does not go away with time.
- Methylprednisolone may cause changes in insulin requirements if your animal is diabetic. You should ask your veterinarian for instructions on how to deal with these changes if your animal is receiving insulin injections.

How Should It Be Given?

- Methylprednisolone and other glucocorticoid drugs should be given orally with food to reduce the chances of stomach ulcers or irritation. If given once daily, prednisone is usually given in the morning to dogs and horses, and in the evening to cats as this will more closely mimic their natural hormone cycles.
- The successful outcome of your animal's treatment with this medication depends upon your commitment and ability to administer it exactly as the veterinarian has prescribed. Please do not skip doses or stop giving the medication. If you have difficulty giving doses consult your veterinarian or pharmacist who can offer administration techniques or change the dosage form to a type of medication that may be more acceptable to you and your animal.
- If you miss a dose of this medication you should give it as soon as you remember it, but if it is within a few hours of the regularly scheduled dose, wait and give it at the regular time. Do not double a dose as this can be toxic to your pet.

- Some other drugs can interact with this medication so tell your veterinarian about any drugs or foods that you currently give your animal. Do not give new foods or medications without first asking your veterinarian.
- **Dogs and Cats**: Dogs and cats usually receive methylprednisolone orally once to twice daily. Dogs usually receive prednisone in the morning and cats usually receive it in the evening if only given once daily as this will more closely mimic their natural hormone cycles. Your veterinarian, may prescribe a tapering (reducing) dose of this medication. More medication is given early in therapy and the dose is slowly tapered. If you have any questions on how much or how often to give this medication, consult with your veterinarian or pharmacist. Some veterinarians will give a long acting form of methylprednisolone injection under the skin every few weeks at the veterinary clinic.
- **Horses**: Horses generally do not receive long term glucocorticoid therapy, but if they do, they receive it orally once daily mixed in the feed. Prednisolone is a better choice than prednisone when given orally to horses. Prednisolone and prednisone are considered Class 4 drugs by the Association of Racing Commissioners International (ARCI).

What Other Information Is Important About This Medication?

- Methylprednisolone should be stored at room temperature in a tight, light resistant, childproof container away from all children and other household pets.
- The injectable sodium succinate form must not be used after 48 hours from the time of reconstituting (making a solution from the powder).
- The injectable suspension for administration in the muscle or under the skin should be shaken well before use.

Metoclopramide

Reglan® is another name for this medication.

How Is This Medication Useful?

- Metoclopramide is used to stimulate the stomach to prevent vomiting as well as help move food and hairballs from the stomach into the intestines. It is not useful in treating constipation, however, as it has little effect on the colon or large intestines.
- It is also useful in preventing stomach acid from backing up into the throat (esophageal reflux).
- Metoclopramide has also been used to prevent the vomiting associated with cancer chemotherapy.

Are There Conditions or Times When Its Use Might Cause More Harm Than Good?

- Metoclopramide and drugs like it should not be used in animals that are allergic to it. Metoclopramide is very similar to the sunscreen agent, PABA, and humans allergic to sunscreens should avoid contact with metoclo-pramide.
- Metoclopramide should not be given to animals who have a stomach blockage, stomach bleeding or have a blockage in the intestines.
- Metoclopramide should not be used in animals that have ever had seizures as it may increase the risk of having another seizure.
- Metoclopramide should not be given to animals with a tumor known as pheochromocytoma as this drug may cause a fatal increase in blood pressure.
- If your animal has any of the above conditions, talk to your veterinarian about the potential risks of using the medication versus the benefits that it might have.

What Side Effects Can Be Seen With Its Use?

- Metoclopramide has very few side effects, but the most common side effects seen are constipation, behavior and attitude changes.
- Some dogs and cats may get very frenzied and disoriented.
- If injected into the veins of horses very fast, metoclopramide can cause severe stomach pain and frenzied behavior. This side effect is not generally seen with oral doses of metoclopramide in horses.

How Should It Be Given?

- Metoclopramide may be given as an injection by your veterinarian or as oral tablets and liquid to be given three times daily.
- The successful outcome of your animal's treatment with this medication depends upon your commitment and ability to administer it exactly as the veterinarian has prescribed. Please do not skip doses or stop giving the medication. If you have difficulty giving doses consult your veterinarian or pharmacist who can offer administration techniques or change the dosage form to a type of medication that may be more acceptable to you and your animal.
- If you miss a dose of this medication you should give it as soon as you remember it, but if it is within a few hours of the regularly scheduled dose, wait and give it at the regular time. Do not double a dose as this can be toxic to your pet.
- Some other drugs can interact with this medication so tell your veterinarian about any drugs or foods that you currently give your animal. Do not give new foods or medications without first asking your veterinarian.
- **Dogs and Cats**: Dogs and cats usually receive metoclopramide tablets or syrup orally three to four times daily. Sometimes metoclopramide injection will be sent home with an owner for injection underneath the skin of the pet.
- **Horses**: Horses generally only receive metoclopramide as a slow injection into the vein in the veterinary clinic. Metoclopramide is an ARCI (Association of Racing Commissioners International) Class 4 drug.

What Other Information Is Important About This Medication?

- Metoclopramide tablets, syrup and injection should be stored in a tight, light resistant, child-proof container away from all children and other household pets.
- Metoclopramide is considered a Class 4 drug under the Uniform Classification Guidelines for the Association of Racing Commissioners International.

Metronidazole

Flagyl®, Metrogel®, and Protostat® are other names for this medication.

How Is This Medication Useful?

- Metronidazole is an antibiotic used to kill intestinal parasites in animals (*e.g.*, giardia). It is also used to treat bacterial infections caused by bacteria known as anaerobes. There are two forms of this drug: metronidazole hydrochloride and metronidazole benzoate. The benzoate form is much less bitter tasting than the hydrochloride form, but benzoate may cause problems if used for very long periods in cats.

Are There Conditions or Times When Its Use Might Cause More Harm Than Good?

- Metronidazole and drugs like it are banned for use in animals that will be used for human food.
- Metronidazole and drugs like it should not be used in animals that are known to be allergic to these drugs.
- Metronidazole should not be used in animals that are pregnant or nursing or in animals that are debilitated in any way. Metronidazole has caused birth defects in laboratory animals, especially early in pregnancy.
- Metronidazole makes it very difficult for the body to process alcohols. You should tell your veterinarian about any liquid medications that you give your pet and not allow your pet to ingest any alcoholic drinks while on this medication.
- Metronidazole can be very toxic to the liver and should probably not be used in animals with liver disease. If metronidazole must be used in these animals, the veterinarian will usually use a much lower dose.
- You should always give all of the medication as directed by your veterinarian. If the entire course of treatment is not finished, the germ causing the infection may become stronger than the antibiotics and cause a worsening infection.
- If your animal has any of the above conditions, talk to your veterinarian about the potential risks of using the medication versus the benefits that it might have.

What Side Effects Can Be Seen With Its Use?

- Side effects reported in animals include nausea, vomiting, weakness, anemia, liver damage, blood in the urine, loss of appetite and diarrhea.

- Damage to the nerves is also a possible side effect and some animals will have seizures as a result. If you see your animal stumbling, knuckling over on its paws, or appearing weak, you should contact your veterinarian immediately.

How Should It Be Given?

- Metronidazole is given oralliy as tablets and liquid, once to twice daily.
- The successful outcome of your animal's treatment with this medication depends upon your commitment and ability to administer it exactly as the veterinarian has prescribed. Please do not skip doses or stop giving the medication. If you have difficulty giving doses consult your veterinarian or pharmacist who can offer administration techniques or change the dosage form to a type of medication that may be more acceptable to you and your animal.
- If you miss a dose of this medication you should give it as soon as you remember it, but if it is within a few hours of the regularly scheduled dose, wait and give it at the regular time. Do not double a dose as this can be toxic to your pet.
- Some other drugs can interact with this medication so tell your veterinarian about any drugs or foods that you currently give your animal. Do not give new foods or medications without first asking your veterinarian.
- **Dogs and Cats**: Dogs and cats usually receive metronidazole orally once or twice daily with food as a liquid or a tablet. Tablets should not be crushed or chewed as they have an extremely bitter taste and will cause your pet to drool and refuse more doses.
- **Horses**: Horses receive metronidazole orally twice to three times daily.

What Other Information Is Important About This Medication?

- Metronidazole should be stored in a tight, light resistant, childproof container away from all children and other household pets.
- Oral liquids should be shaken well and stored in the refrigerator.
- Metronidazole should never be used in animals that may be used for human food.

VETERINARY DRUG HANDBOOK-Client Information Edition
Permission to photocopy for individual clients granted by Gigi Davidson and Donald C. Plumb © 2003

Milbemycin

Interceptor® is another name for this medication.

How Is This Medication Useful?

- Milbemycin is a drug used to prevent heartworm disease, certain intestinal worms, and to treat certain kinds of mange.

Are There Conditions or Times When Its Use Might Cause More Harm Than Good?

- Milbemycin should not be used in animals that are allergic to it or to drugs like it.
- If your pet has a large amount of immature heartworms (microfilaria) in its blood, milbemycin may cause them to all die off at once and cause a very serious reaction in your pet. Your veterinarian will want to do a heartworm test on your pet before starting milbemycin.
- Milbemycin does get into the milk of nursing mothers, but it has not caused any problems in babies nursing milk from mothers who are taking milbemycin.
- If you are stopping the once daily heartworm prevention, then you must start milbemycin within 30 days or your pet may get heartworms.
- At higher doses, milbemycin may get into the brains of Collies and other herding breeds and cause coma and even death. If your pet shows any sign of weakness, confusion or stumbling, notify your veterinarian immediately.
- Milbemycin tablets are flavored with a pork liver extract and may cause food allergies in some patients.
- You should not use milbemycin in animals less than 8 weeks old.
- If your animal has any of the above conditions, talk to your veterinarian about the potential risks of using the medication versus the benefits that it might have.

What Side Effects Can Be Seen With Its Use?

- Milbemycin may cause a serious reaction in pets with high amounts of immature heartworms in their blood. Your veterinarian will do a heartworm test on your pet before prescribing milbemycin.
- Milbemycin at high doses can get into the brains of some animals and cause damage. If you notice that your pet is stumbling, weak, confused, or shows any signs of behavior change, you should notify your veterinarian immediately.

How Should It Be Given?

- The successful outcome of your animal's treatment with this medication depends upon your commitment and ability to administer it exactly as the veterinarian has prescribed. Please do not skip doses or stop giving the medication. If you have difficulty giving doses consult your veterinarian or pharmacist who can offer administration techniques or change the dosage form to a type of medication that may be more acceptable to you and your animal.
- If you miss a dose of this medication you should give it as soon as you remember it, but if it is within a few hours of the regularly scheduled dose, wait and give it at the regular time. Do not double a dose as this can be toxic to your pet. If you miss more than 8 weeks of giving this drug, you should have your pet tested for hearworms within 6 months as they may have become infected during the time the drug was not given.
- Some other drugs can interact with this medication so tell your veterinarian about any drugs or foods that you currently give your animal. Do not give new foods or medications without first asking your veterinarian.
- **Dogs and Cats**: Milbemycin is usually given orally to dogs and cats once monthly for heartworm prevention. Milbemycin may be given orally once daily to dogs with certain kinds of mange.

What Other Information Is Important About This Medication?

- Milbemycin should be stored in a tight, light resistant, childproof container away from all children and other household pets.

Permission to photocopy for individual clients granted by Gigi Davidson and Donald C. Plumb © 2003

Misoprostol

Cytotec® is another name for this medication.

How Is This Medication Useful?

- Misoprostol is used to help heal stomach ulcers and protect against ulcers caused by some drugs. Misoprostol is also used with other drugs to help control allergic skin disease in dogs. It has also been given to animals to protect kidneys from damage caused by a drug called cyclosporine.

Are There Conditions or Times When Its Use Might Cause More Harm Than Good?

- Misoprostol can cause miscarriage. It should not be handled by pregnant women and should not be given to pregnant animals.
- Misoprostel enters mother's milk and can cause serious diarrhea in nursing offspring.
- Misoprostol should not be used in animals that have problems with the blood vessels in their brain or hearts as these animals may suffer seizures or a dangerous drop in blood pressure. If your animal has a history of seizures or a problem with blood vessels you should tell your veterinarian.
- If your animal has any of the above conditions, talk to your veterinarian about the potential risks of using the medication versus the benefits that it might have.

What Side Effects Can Be Seen With Its Use?

- The most common side effect of misoprostol is stomach upset with diarrhea and vomiting. Some animals will have excessive gas. Usually these side effects will go away in a few days. Giving misoprostol with food may also lessen these side effects.
- Some female animals will experience uterine cramps and bleeding from the vagina. If your animal experiences these side effects, contact your veterinarian for advice.

How Should It Be Given?

- Misoprostol should be given with food orally three times daily. Pregnant women should not handle this drug at all and should have another family member give the drug to the pet.
- The successful outcome of your animal's treatment with this medication depends upon your commitment and ability to administer it exactly as the veterinarian has prescribed. Please do not skip doses or stop giving the medication. If you have difficulty giving doses consult your veterinarian or pharmacist who can offer administration techniques or change the dosage form to a type of medication that may be more acceptable to you and your animal.
- If you miss a dose of this medication you should give it as soon as you remember it, but if it is within a few hours of the regularly scheduled dose, wait and give it at the regular time. Do not double a dose as this can be toxic to your pet.
- Some other drugs can interact with this medication so tell your veterinarian about any drugs or foods that you currently give your animal. Do not give new foods or medications without first asking your veterinarian.
- **Dogs and Cats**: Dogs and cats usually receive misoprostol orally with food three times daily. Pregnant animals should not receive this drug.
- **Horses**: Horses may receive this drug orally three times daily.

What Other Information Is Important About This Medication?

- Misoprostol should be stored in a tight, light resistant, childproof container away from all children and other household pets.
- Misoprostol can cause miscarriage and should not be handled by pregnant women or given to pregnant animals.

Mitotane

Lysodren® or o,p-DDD are other names for this medication.

How Is This Medication Useful?

- Mitotane stops the growth of cells in the adrenal gland. In animals it is used to treat Cushing's Disease (adrenal glands produce too much cortisol).

Are There Conditions or Times When Its Use Might Cause More Harm Than Good?

- Mitotane should not be used in animals that are allergic to it or to drugs like it.
- Mitotane should not be used in pregnant animals. It should also not be handled by women who are pregnant or are trying to get pregnant.
- Mitotane may alter the insulin requirements of diabetic patients. If your pet is diabetic, your veterinarian may need to readjust your pet's insulin doses.
- Mitotane is eliminated from the body by the kidneys and liver; animals with severe liver or kidney disease should probably not receive mitotane.
- Mitotane decreases the body's ability to handle stress. Your veterinarian will give you some prednisone or prednisolone to help your animal get through stressful periods (household guests, new babies, new pets, travel, injury, surgery, illness, etc.).
- If your animal has any of the above conditions, talk to your veterinarian about the potential risks of using the medication versus the benefits that it might have.

What Side Effects Can Be Seen With Its Use?

- The most common side effects are stomach upset, diarrhea and vomiting. Most animals will get more tired when the mitotane is starting to work. Mitotane must be given in big doses until it starts to work in your dog. Most dogs will have an effect within 5-14days after which your veterinarian will reduce the dose from giving it twice daily to giving it twice a week. Some animals take as little as 2 days to respond while others may take as much as 35 days. If your animal becomes unusually tired or weak, you should contact your veterinarian immediately so that he may determine the cause of the weakness and adjust the dose of mitotane if needed.

- Some animals may develop liver problems from mitotane. If your animal stops eating, acts unusually tired, or has a yellowish color to its gums and the whites of its eyes, you should contact your veterinarian immediately.
- Mitotane may alter the doses of insulin in diabetic patients.
- Mitotane may alter the doses of drugs used to control epilepsy.

How Should It Be Given?

- Mitotane should be given orally with an oily or fatty food. Mitotane liquids and powders sprinkled on food with a little corn oil are the best ways to give mitotane to your pet. But if your pet has been controlled on intact tablets for a long time, you should not start crushing the tablets or switch to a liquid form without talking to your veterinarian. Switching from tablets to oral liquids or powders will dramatically increase the amount of mitotane that gets into your pet's bloodstream.
- Mitotane is usually prescribed at high doses for 1-2 weeks until it has an effect. After that time, mitotane doses are usually given only two times a week.
- You can tell if mitotane is starting to work when your animal drinks less, eats less, and urinates less. If you are not sure how much water your pet drinks, you should offer water in a measuring bowl or draw lines on the water bowl so that you can tell water intake has decreased.
- Your veterinarian will usually give you a drug called prednisone or prednisolone to help your animal through periods of stress. If you travel, have house guests, get a new pet or your animal gets sick or hurt, you should contact your veterinarian for instructions on how much prednisone to give during these times.
- Humans should avoid contact with mitotane and should wear gloves while handling it. Hands should always be washed after handling.
- Pregnant women should not handle mitotane.

(Continued on following page)

Mitotane

How Should It Be Given? (continued from previous page)

- The successful outcome of your animal's treatment with this medication depends upon your commitment and ability to administer it exactly as the veterinarian has prescribed. Please do not skip doses or stop giving the medication. If you have difficulty giving doses consult your veterinarian or pharmacist who can offer administration techniques or change the dosage form to a type of medication that may be more acceptable to you and your animal.

- If you miss a dose of this medication you should give it as soon as you remember it, but if it is within a few hours of the regularly scheduled dose, wait and give it at the regular time. Do not double a dose as this can be toxic to your pet.

- Some other drugs can interact with this medication so tell your veterinarian about any drugs or foods that you currently give your animal. Do not give new foods or medications without first asking your veterinarian.

- **Dogs and Cats**: Dogs usually receive mitotane orally twice daily initially (loading period) and then twice weekly once they respond to mitotane therapy. Cats do not usually receive mitotane.

- **Ferrets**: Ferrets may receive mitotane orally for Cushing's disease or for certain tumors that did not respond to surgery.

What Other Information Is Important About This Medication?

- Mitotane should be stored in a tight, light resistant, childproof container away from all children and other household pets.

- Gloves should always be worn when handling this drug and hands washed afterwards.

- Mitotane should not be allowed into the soil and water as it can be very damaging to the environment. Any leftover drug should be returned to your veterinarian or pharmacist for proper disposal.

VETERINARY DRUG HANDBOOK-Client Information Edition
Permission to photocopy for individual clients granted by Gigi Davidson and Donald C. Plumb © 2003

Morphine Sulfate

How Is This Medication Useful?

- Morphine is a narcotic that is useful to treat moderate to severe pain, especially in dogs. It has also been used to treat severe cough or diarrhea.
- Use of oral sustained release tablets is increasingly being used by veterinarians to reduce pain associated with cancer or other causes.

Are There Conditions or Times When Its Use Might Cause More Harm Than Good?

- Morphine should not be used in animals who are hypersensitive to it or other opiate drugs (codeine, etc).
- Morphine should not be given to animals who are receiving drugs known as MAO inhibitors (Mitaban® Dip, Preventic® Flea Collars, Anipryl®, and isoniazid are a few of these drugs). Aged cheese can also cause this effect, so make sure that your pets do not get into any aged cheese while on this drug.
- It should be used with caution in dogs or cats with thyroid, heart, kidney, liver, lung, or adrenal gland diseases.
- Patients with head injuries, and old or debilitated animals should also receive the drug with caution.
- It must not be used in animals with diarrhea caused by a toxic substance, until that substance has been eliminated.
- Working dogs (e.g., guide dogs, search dogs, hunting dogs, sled dogs, rescue dogs) may become overly sedated and unable to perform their duties while on this drug.
- Horses may become overly stimulated when receiving morphine by injection and it should be administered by injection only by a veterinarian.
- If your animal has any of the above conditions, talk to your veterinarian about the potential risks of using the medication versus the benefits that it might have.

What Side Effects Can Be Seen With Its Use?

- The most common side effect in dogs is sedation. Most animals will become tolerant to this effect with time and the sleepiness will wear off.
- Morphine can cause a variety of gastrointestinal effects, including vomiting, decreased appetite, and constipation. Dogs may defecate suddenly and unexpectedly after receiving the first dose of morphine. Make sure your dog has access to the outdoors when giving the first dose of morphine, or at least make sure it is laying on a washable or disposable pad in case your pet has an accident.
- Morphine depresses breathing function which may cause problems in susceptible animals.
- Dogs may develop low body temperature and cats may experience increased body temperature while receiving morphine
- Cats may become unusually excited while taking this drug and tremors and seizures have been noted.

How Should It Be Given?

- The successful outcome of your animal's treatment with this medication depends upon your commitment and ability to administer it exactly as the veterinarian has prescribed. If you have difficulty giving any doses, please do not skip doses or stop giving the medication.
- Consult your veterinarian or pharmacist who can offer administration techniques or change the dosage form to a type of medication that may be more acceptable to you and your animal.
- If your veterinarian has prescribed this drug to be used routinely and you miss a dose, you should give it as soon as you remember it, but wait the appropriate amount of time before giving the following doses. Do not double a dose as this can be toxic to your pet.
- Some other drugs can interact with this medication so tell your veterinarian about any drugs or foods that you currently give your animal. Do not give new foods or medications without first asking your veterinarian.
- **Dogs and cats**: Dogs and cats usually receive morphine orally two to six times daily depending on their degree of pain. Do not give your pet aged cheese or use tick collars while on this drug.
- **Horses** do not usually receive morphine orally as it can stop the intestines and lead to colic.

What Other Information Is Important About This Medication?

- Morphine is a controlled substance and should not be given to anyone other than the animal for whom it was prescribed. It is in a very restricted category and your veterinarian will need to write a new prescription each time you fill this prescription..
- Morphine tablets or oral solution should be stored at room temperature in a tight, light resistant, childproof container away from all children and other household pets.
- Morphine is available for injectable use, but it should be given by your veterinarian.

Neomycin Sulfate

Biosol® is another name for this medication.

How Is This Medication Useful?

- Neomycin sulfate is used to kill most of the bacteria in the intestines prior to intestinal surgery. It also is used to kill bacteria in the intestines that can create ammonia and cause problems in the brain and bloodstream when the liver is not working properly.

Are There Conditions or Times When Its Use Might Cause More Harm Than Good?

- Neomycin should not be given to animals who are allergic to it or drugs like it.
- Cats seem to be more allergic to neomycin than other animals and some cats have had fatal allergic reactions after using neomycin products in the eye.
- Neomycin should not be given to animals with a blockage in their stomach or intestines.
- Neomycin and drugs like it can cause an irreversible deafness. This side effect can harm the performance of guide dogs or herding dogs. If you notice that your pet has a head tilt or appears to not be hearing well, you should contact your veterinarian immediately.
- Neomycin and drugs like it can cause severe kidney damage. Neomycin should be used very carefully in very young or very old animals and should not be used at all in animals with kidney damage.
- Neomycin can cause the muscles to not work well and should not be used in animals with muscle disorders such as myasthenia gravis.
- Neomycin and drugs like it can kill all the helpful bacteria in the intestines of rabbits and result in death. Neomycin should not be used in rabbits.
- Neomycin can also cause all of these problems in unborn animals and should not be used in pregnant animals unless it will save the life of the mother.
- If your animal has any of the above conditions, talk to your veterinarian about the potential risks of using the medication versus the benefits that it might have.

What Side Effects Can Be Seen With Its Use?

- Neomycin and drugs like it can cause deafness. If your animal shows any signs of a head tilt, loss of balance, or acts like it is having trouble hearing, you should contact your veterinarian immediately. Cats are more likely to have this side effect than other animals.

- Neomycin can cause kidney damage. If you notice that your animal is urinating more, or acts like it isn't feeling well, you should contact your veterinarian immediately.
- Neomycin can cause muscle weakness. If your animal appears to be stumbling or weak, you should contact your veterinarian immediately.

How Should It Be Given?

- Neomycin is only given by mouth, in the rectum, or as a topical ointment because it causes more kidney damage if given by injection.
- The successful outcome of your animal's treatment with this medication depends upon your commitment and ability to administer it exactly as the veterinarian has prescribed. Please do not skip doses or stop giving the medication. If you have difficulty giving doses consult your veterinarian or pharmacist who can offer administration techniques or change the dosage form to a type of medication that may be more acceptable to you and your animal.
- If you miss a dose of this medication you should give it as soon as you remember it, but if it is within a few hours of the regularly scheduled dose, wait and give it at the regular time. Do not double a dose as this can be toxic to your pet.
- Some other drugs can interact with this medication so tell your veterinarian about any drugs or foods that you currently give your animal. Do not give new foods or medications without first asking your veterinarian.
- **Dogs and Cats**: Dogs and cats usually receive neomycin as an oral liquid three to four times daily.
- **Horses**: Adult horses may receive neomycin as a liquid three to four times daily. It should probably not be given to foals.
- **Rabbits**: Neomycin should not be used in rabbits as it may kill them.

What Other Information Is Important About This Medication?

- Neomycin should be stored in a tight, light resistant, childproof container away from all children and other household pets.
- Allergic reactions to neomycin can be fatal in cats. If your cat starts to act itchy, have swelling of the face, tongue or throat, or has difficulty breathing, you should get it to the nearest veterinary clinic immediately.

VETERINARY DRUG HANDBOOK-Client Information Edition

Omeprazole

Gastrogard®, Prilosec® and Nexium® are other names for this medication.

How Is This Medication Useful?

- Omeprazole is a medication that is used to treat stomach ulcers as well as to prevent the formation of stomach ulcers. It works by reducing the amount of acid that enters the stomach.

Are There Conditions or Times When Its Use Might Cause More Harm Than Good?

- Animals allergic to omeprazole or to drugs like it should not receive this drug.
- As omeprazole is removed from the body by the liver and kidneys, it should be used with caution in animals with liver and kidney disease or the drug may become toxic.
- It is not known whether omeprazole can be used safely in pregnant animals. Some laboratory animals have shown a higher rate of miscarriage when high doses of omeprazole are given. It should probably only be used in pregnant or nursing mothers if it will save the life of the mother.
- If your animal has any of the above conditions, talk to your veterinarian about the potential risks of using the medication versus the benefits that it might have.

What Side Effects Can Be Seen With Its Use?

- There are few side effects from omeprazole. It may cause a rash in some animals.
- Some animals may develop stomach ache, vomiting and diarrhea, and excessive gas. If your animal develops any of these side effects, you should contact your veterinarian.
- Some humans have developed anemia while taking this drug, but it is not know if this effect occurs in animals.
- Because of some possible links to cancer when used in lab animals, omeprazole is generally not used for longer than 4 weeks in dogs and cats and 90 days in horses. If the benefits outweigh the risks, however, it may be given for longer.

How Should It Be Given?

- Omeprazole capsules should be given unopened. If your veterinarian has instructed you to give omeprazole capsules as a liquid, you should be very careful when handling the beads inside the capsules and only mix it with fruit juices. It should not be mixed with water or milk as these will destroy the protective covering on the beads.
- The paste for horses should be given as directed by the veterinarian. The person giving the paste should pay attention to the marks on the handle of the tube. If you are not giving whole tubes of paste each dose, your veterinarian will show you exactly where to dial the ring on the tube to avoid over-dosing your horse.
- The successful outcome of your animal's treatment with this medication depends upon your commitment and ability to administer it exactly as the veterinarian has prescribed. Please do not skip doses or stop giving the medication. If you have difficulty giving doses consult your veterinarian or pharmacist who can offer administration techniques or change the dosage form to a type of medication that may be more acceptable to you and your animal.
- If you miss a dose of this medication you should give it as soon as you remember it, but if it is within a few hours of the regularly scheduled dose, wait and give it at the regular time. Do not double a dose as this can be toxic to your pet.
- Some other drugs can interact with this medication so tell your veterinarian about any drugs or foods that you currently give your animal. Do not give new foods or medications without first asking your veterinarian.
- **Dogs and Cats**: Dogs and cats usually receive this medication orally once daily.
- **Horses**: Horses usually receive this drug orally once daily for a month while treating ulcers. Some horses will receive omeprazole for one more month at a lower dose to prevent the ulcers from coming back.

What Other Information Is Important About This Medication?

- Omeprazole should be stored in a tight, light resistant, childproof container away from all children and other household pets. It should never be stored at temperatures higher than 86°F, so you should keep it indoors during the hot part of summer or in climates where the temperature exceeds 86°F. The barn is generally not a good place to store drugs.
- Omeprazole is considered a Class 5 drug by the Association of Racing Commissioners International.

Ondansetron

Zofran® is another name for this medication.

How Is This Medication Useful?

- Ondansetron is a drug that stops or prevents severe vomiting such as that seen with chemotherapy. Animals who have been given ondansetron for severe vomiting seem to be much more relaxed and comfortable within 15 minutes of getting the drug. It is one of the strongest anti-vomiting drugs available, but because of its great expense, is usually used only when other drugs have failed to stop vomiting.

Are There Conditions or Times When Its Use Might Cause More Harm Than Good?

- Ondansetron may mask the symptoms of a stomach or intestinal blockage or stoppage.
- As ondansetron is removed from the body by the liver, it should be used very carefully in animals that have liver disease as the drug may become toxic to your pet.
- Collies and some other herding breeds may be very sensitive to ondansetron and may have severe side effects from this drug.
- If your animal has any of the above conditions, talk to your veterinarian about the potential risks of using the medication versus the benefits that it might have.

What Side Effects Can Be Seen With Its Use?

- Ondansetron has very few side effects at normal doses. It may cause constipation.
- Rarely in humans, it has caused irregular heart beat, low blood pressure, and jerky movements of the muscles. It is not known if it has these same effects in animal patients.

How Should It Be Given?

- Ondansetron is usually given orally once to twice daily. It may also be given by injection by your veterinarian just prior to giving chemotherapy at the veterinary clinic.
- If your veterinarian prescribes the topical gel form of ondansetron, you should make sure that you wear gloves when applying it to your pet.

- The successful outcome of your animal's treatment with this medication depends upon your commitment and ability to administer it exactly as the veterinarian has prescribed. Please do not skip doses or stop giving the medication. If you have difficulty giving doses consult your veterinarian or pharmacist who can offer administration techniques or change the dosage form to a type of medication that may be more acceptable to you and your animal.
- If you miss a dose of this medication you should give it as soon as you remember it, but if it is within a few hours of the regularly scheduled dose, wait and give it at the regular time. Do not double a dose as this can be toxic to your pet.
- Some other drugs can interact with this medication so tell your veterinarian about any drugs or foods that you currently give your animal. Do not give new foods or medications without first asking your veterinarian.
- **Dogs and Cats**: Dogs and cats usually receive this drug as an injection in the veterinary clinic. It may also be given orally once to three times daily. As animals with severe vomiting do not keep medication on the stomach very well, ondansetron has also been compounded by pharmacists into a gel that can be rubbed on the skin to stop vomiting.
- **Horses**: Due to the great expense of ondansetron, it is not usually given to horses.

What Other Information Is Important About This Medication?

- Ondansetron should be stored in a tight, light resistant, childproof container away from all children and other household pets.
- Ondansetron is very expensive, but also very effective in stopping vomiting.

Orbifloxacin

Orbax® is another name for this medication.

How Is This Medication Useful?

- Orbifloxacin is a quinolone antibiotic used to treat infections in animals.

Are There Conditions or Times When Its Use Might Cause More Harm Than Good?

- Animals allergic to orbifloxacin or drugs like it should not receive orbifloxacin.
- Orbifloxacin and drugs like it should not be used in animals that are still growing because it may affect joints and bone growth. Some infections are serious enough, however, that you and your veterinarian may wish to risk this effect.
- Orbifloxacin and drugs like it can cause blindness in cats. Your veterinarian will prescribe orbifloxacin at a safe dose, but if your cat shows any signs of dilated pupils or any change in behavior, you should contact your veterinarian immediately. Orbifloxacin is not as likely to cause this effect as a drug called enrofloxacin (Baytri®).
- Orbifloxacin and other quinolones may rarely cause a seizure in animals that are prone to seizures. If your pet has ever had a seizure, you should tell your veterinarian before administering orbifloxacin.
- Orbifloxacin is forbidden to be used in any animal that will be used as food for humans.
- You should always give all of the medication as directed by your veterinarian. If the entire course of treatment is not finished, the germ causing the infection may become stronger than the antibiotics and cause a worsening infection.
- If your animal has any of the above conditions, talk to your veterinarian about the potential risks of using the medication versus the benefits that it might have.

What Side Effects Can Be Seen With Its Use?

- Except for the effects mentioned above, orbifloxacin is generally free of any side effects. Some animals will suffer from loss of appetite, vomiting, diarrhea, and tiredness.
- Rarely, some animals will develop liver problems after taking orbifloxacin.
- Dehydrated animals who are prone to seizures, may have seizures while taking orbifloxacin.

How Should It Be Given?

- Orbifloxacin should be given orally on an empty stomach. Iron, antacids and dairy products should not be given within 2 hours after giving orbifloxacin.
- The successful outcome of your animal's treatment with this medication depends upon your commitment and ability to administer it exactly as the veterinarian has prescribed. Do not stop giving the antibiotics just because your pet looks better. Please do not skip doses or stop giving the medication. If you have difficulty giving doses consult your veterinarian or pharmacist who can offer administration techniques or change the dosage form to a type of medication that may be more acceptable to you and your animal.
- Giving antibiotics irregularly can actually make the infection worse as the bacteria can build up a tolerance to the drug (resistance).
- If you miss a dose of this medication you should give it as soon as you remember it, but if it is within a few hours of the regularly scheduled dose, wait and give it at the regular time. Do not double a dose as this can be toxic to your pet.
- Some other drugs can interact with this medication so tell your veterinarian about any drugs or foods that you currently give your animal. Do not give new foods or medications without first asking your veterinarian.
- **Dogs and Cats**: Dogs and cats usually receive orbifloxacin orally once to twice daily for several days.
- **Horses**: Horses generally do not receive orbifloxacin but may receive it orally once daily mixed with feed.

What Other Information Is Important About This Medication?

- Orbifloxacin should be stored in a tight, light resistant, childproof container away from all children and other household pets.

Oxazepam

Serax® is another name for this medication.

How Is This Medication Useful?

- Oxazepam is a drug similar to diazepam (Valium®), but is used in animals primarily as an appetite stimulant in cats

Are There Conditions or Times When Its Use Might Cause More Harm Than Good?

- Oxazepam should not be given to any animal that is allergic to it or drugs like it (e.g., diazepam/Valium®).
- As oxazepam is cleared from the body by the liver, it should be used carefully in animals with liver disease.
- Rarely, in humans this drug has caused a type of seizure, so it should be used with caution in animals with seizure disorders.
- Oxazepam safety in pregnancy or in nursing animals is not known.
- If your animal has any of the above conditions, talk to your veterinarian about the potential risks of using the medication versus the benefits that it might have.

What Side Effects Can Be Seen With Its Use?

- The usual effects are drowsiness and sedation.
- Cats may develop incoordination and difficulty breathing at higher doses.

How Should It Be Given?

- The successful outcome of your animal's treatment with this medication depends upon your commitment and ability to administer it exactly as the veterinarian has prescribed. Please do not skip doses or stop giving the medication. If you have difficulty giving doses consult your veterinarian or pharmacist who can offer administration techniques or change the dosage form to a type of medication that may be more acceptable to you and your animal.

- Some other drugs can interact with this medication so tell your veterinarian about any drugs or foods that you currently give your animal. Do not give new foods or medications without first asking your veterinarian.
- If you miss a dose of this medication you should give it as soon as you remember it, but if it is within a few hours of the regularly scheduled dose, wait and give it at the regular time. Do not double a dose as this can be toxic to your pet.
- **Dogs and Cats**: Cats usually receive this medication twice daily by mouth. Dogs usually don't receive this medication.
- **Horses**: Horses do not generally receive oxazepam.

What Other Information Is Important About This Medication?

- Oxazepam capsules or tablets should be stored at room temperature and protected from light and moisture.
- Because the usual dosage for a cat is 2 mg, and the smallest commercially available strength is 10 mg; your veterinarian may prescribe a dosage form that will be made by your pharmacist.
- Oxazepam is a controlled substance and you will need to get a new prescription every 6 months if your pet is on long term therapy.
- You should not give oxazepam to any other pets or household members.

Oxybutynin

Ditropan® is another name for this medication.

How Is This Medication Useful?

- Oxybutynin is used to stop spasms of the bladder which cause leaking of urine from the bladder.

Are There Conditions or Times When Its Use Might Cause More Harm Than Good?

- Oxybutynin should not be used if your pet has a stomach or an intestinal blockage or stoppage.
- Oxybutynin should not be used in patients that have myasthenia gravis or heart disease.
- Oxybutynin should not be used in animals that have overactive thyroid, glaucoma, overactive bowels (colitis), inability to urinate, or kidney stones. The effects of this drug may worsen these conditions.
- If your animal has any of the above conditions, talk to your veterinarian about the potential risks of using the medication versus the benefits that it might have.

What Side Effects Can Be Seen With Its Use?

- Oxybutynin may cause the following side effects in your pet: diarrhea or constipation, inability to urinate, drooling and sleepiness.
- Some animals will have a dry mouth, fast heartbeat, lose their appetite, vomiting, weakness, or dilated pupils.
- If too much oxybutynin has been given (overdose) your pet may show signs of restlessness, excitement, fast heartbeat, fever, or seizures. If your pet shows any of these signs, contact your veterinarian immediately.

How Should It Be Given?

- The successful outcome of your animal's treatment with this medication depends upon your commitment and ability to administer it exactly as the veterinarian has prescribed. Please do not skip doses or stop giving the medication. If you have difficulty giving doses consult your veterinarian or pharmacist who can offer administration techniques or change the dosage form to a type of medication that may be more acceptable to you and your animal.
- If you miss a dose of this medication you should give it as soon as you remember it, but if it is within a few hours of the regularly scheduled dose, wait and give it at the regular time. Do not double a dose as this can be toxic to your pet.
- Some other drugs can interact with this medication so tell your veterinarian about any drugs or foods that you currently give your animal. Do not give new foods or medications without first asking your veterinarian.
- **Dogs and Cats**: Dogs and cats usually receive this drug orally two to three times daily. It may be given once or twice daily in younger animals.
- **Horses**: This medication is generally not given to horses due to the risk of colic.

What Other Information Is Important About This Medication?

- Oxybutynin should be stored in a tight, light resistant, childproof container away from all children and other household pets.

Pancrelipase

Pancrezyme® and Viokase® are other names for this medication.

How Is This Medication Useful?

- Pancrelipase is a collection of secretions (enzymes) from the pancreas that are given to animals whose pancreas has stopped functioning. These enzymes are necessary to help your pet digest fat, protein and sugars in its diet. As pets that do not properly digest their food get diarrhea, pancrelipase helps digest food and stop diarrhea. It is also given to animals such as rabbits and cats to help digest fur balls.

Are There Conditions or Times When Its Use Might Cause More Harm Than Good?

- Since pancrelipase is collected from pig pancreas, it should not be used in animals that have shown an allergy to pork products. Talk to your veterinarian about the potential risks of using the medication versus the benefits that it might have if your animal has pork sensitivity.
- Inhalation of the powder will cause irritation of the lungs and throat and may trigger an asthma attack. Do not inhale this powder or let your pet inhale the powder.
- It will also burn skin on contact. Wash immediately if you get any on your skin or your pet's skin.

What Side Effects Can Be Seen With Its Use?

- High doses may cause diarrhea, vomiting, excessive gas and stomach cramping.

How Should It Be Given?

- Pancrelipase is usually most effective when given as a powder. It is also available in capsules and tablets.
- Pancrelipase should be mixed on the food and left to stand for 15-20 minutes before feeding. This gives the drug a chance to digest nutrients that are helpful to your pet.
- Once your pet's diarrhea gets better, your veterinarian may have you try decreasing the dose to the least amount that prevents diarrhea and allows your pet to gain weight.

- The successful outcome of your animal's treatment with this medication depends upon your commitment and ability to administer it exactly as the veterinarian has prescribed. Please do not skip doses or stop giving the medication. If you have difficulty giving doses consult your veterinarian or pharmacist who can offer administration techniques or change the dosage form to a type of medication that may be more acceptable to you and your animal.
- If you miss a dose of this medication you should give it as soon as you remember it, but if it is within a few hours of the regularly scheduled dose, wait and give it at the regular time. Do not double a dose as this can be toxic to your pet.
- Some other drugs can interact with this medication so tell your veterinarian about any drugs or foods that you currently give your animal. Do not give new foods or medications without first asking your veterinarian.
- **Dogs and Cats:** Dogs and cats usually receive pancrelipase that has been mixed with food and left to stand for 15-20 minutes before feeding.
- **Horses:** Horses do not usually receive pancrelipase enzymes because their diet is very different from dogs and cats and they do not require these enzymes for digestion.
- **Rabbits:** Rabbits may get pancrelipase powder mixed in yogurt to help dissolve fur balls.

What Other Information Is Important About This Medication?

- Pancrelipase should be stored in a tight, light resistant, childproof container away from all children and other household pets.
- Because it is a strong digestive enzyme, it will irritate and burn your skin. If you get it on your skin or the pet's skin, you should wash it off immediately.
- There is also a form of pancrelipase made for humans. It does not contain as much enzymes as the product made for pets. Be sure that you get the right form for your pet.
- Pancrelipase therapy can be very expensive and is usually given for life.

Paroxetine

Paxil® is another name for this medication.

How Is This Medication Useful?

- Paroxetine is a drug used to correct undesirable behavior in animals such as aggression, fear of noises such as thunderstorms, and self-mutilation (pulling fur out or licking skin until it makes a sore.) It may also be used to stop horses from weaving.

Are There Conditions or Times When Its Use Might Cause More Harm Than Good?

- Paroxetine should not be used in animals who are also receiving drugs known as MAO inhibitors (Mitaban® Dip, Preventic® Flea Collars, Anipryl®, and isoniazid are a few of these drugs).. When paroxetine is given with these drugs it can cause serious increases in blood pressure that can cause death. Aged cheese can also cause this effect, so make sure that your pets do not get into any aged cheese while on this drug. If your pet is receiving any of these medications, your veterinarian will ask you to stop giving them for at least 2-5 weeks before prescribing paroxetine.
- Paroxetine should be used with caution in pets that have a history of seizures as it may cause a seizure.
- Paroxetine is removed from the body by the liver and kidneys and should be used very carefully in animals that have liver or kidney disease.
- It is not known if paroxetine can be used safely in pregnancy. It should be used in pregnant animals only when the benefit to the mother outweighs the risk to the babies.
- If your animal has any of the above conditions, talk to your veterinarian about the potential risks of using the medication versus the benefits that it might have.

What Side Effects Can Be Seen With Its Use?

- Paroxetine has not shown many side effects in animals at normal doses. It may cause tiredness, stomach upset, anxiety, restlessness and irritability.
- Loss of appetite is a common side effect of paroxetine in dogs.

How Should It Be Given?

- Paroxetine should be given with or without food orally once daily.
- The successful outcome of your animal's treatment with this medication depends upon your commitment and ability to administer it exactly as the veterinarian has prescribed. Please do not skip doses or stop giving the medication. If you have difficulty giving doses consult your veterinarian or pharmacist who can offer administration techniques or change the dosage form to a type of medication that may be more acceptable to you and your animal.
- If you miss a dose of this medication you should give it as soon as you remember it, but if it is within a few hours of the regularly scheduled dose, wait and give it at the regular time. Do not double a dose as this can be toxic to your pet.
- Some other drugs can interact with this medication so tell your veterinarian about any drugs or foods that you currently give your animal. Do not give new foods or medications without first asking your veterinarian.
- **Dogs and Cats**: Dogs and cats usually receive paroxetine orally once daily. Do not give your pet aged cheese or use tick collars while on this drug.
- **Horses**: Paroxetine has been given orally once daily for horses that are suffering from weaving.

What Other Information Is Important About This Medication?

- Paroxetine should be stored in a tight, light resistant, childproof container away from all children and other household pets.

Pentoxifylline

Trental® is another name for this medication.

How Is This Medication Useful?

- Pentoxifylline is used to increase the life span of red blood cells and increase blood flow to areas that do not get enough blood. Non-healing skin ulcers are an example of this kind of condition. Pentoxifylline is also used to treat the poisons given off in the intestines by bacteria during horse colic (endotoxemia). It is also used for Sickle Cell Anemia in humans.

Are There Conditions or Times When Its Use Might Cause More Harm Than Good?

- Pentoxifylline should not be used in patients that are allergic to it or to drugs like it (amino-phylline, theophylline, caffeine).
- Animals who have or have had bleeding in the brain or eyes should also not receive pentoxifylline. Pentoxifylline should be used very carefully in animals that may be at risk for any kind of excessive bleeding.
- Because pentoxifylline is removed from the body by the liver and kidneys, it should be used very carefully in animals with liver or kidney disease.
- It is not known if pentoxifylline can be used safely in pregnant animals. It also enters the milk, so should not be used in nursing mothers unless the benefit to the mother is greater than the risk to the babies.
- If your animal has any of the above conditions, talk to your veterinarian about the potential risks of using the medication versus the benefits that it might have.

What Side Effects Can Be Seen With Its Use?

- The most common side effect of pentoxifylline is vomiting. Pentoxifylline is in the same drug class as caffeine (coffee). It can cause restlessness, fast heartbeat, dizziness, stomach ache, and even seizures in high doses. This effect may be increased by certain antibiotics known as quinolones.
- If your pet seems unusually restless after receiving pentoxifylline, you should call your veterinarian.

How Should It Be Given?

- Pentoxifylline should be given orally to animals twice to three times daily.
- The human tablets are often too big to give to dogs and cats. Your pharmacist may compound special capsules, medicated treats, or a liquid to give your pet the correct dose. Horses will often receive many of the human tablets as a single dose, and these tablets may be crushed and given with syrup or molasses.
- The successful outcome of your animal's treatment with this medication depends upon your commitment and ability to administer it exactly as the veterinarian has prescribed. Please do not skip doses or stop giving the medication. If you have difficulty giving doses consult your veterinarian or pharmacist who can offer administration techniques or change the dosage form to a type of medication that may be more acceptable to you and your animal.
- If you miss a dose of this medication you should give it as soon as you remember it, but if it is within a few hours of the regularly scheduled dose, wait and give it at the regular time. Do not double a dose as this can be toxic to your pet.
- Some other drugs can interact with this medication so tell your veterinarian about any drugs or foods that you currently give your animal. Do not give new foods or medications without first asking your veterinarian.
- **Dogs and Cats**: Dogs and cats usually receive this medication orally twice to three times daily with food.
- **Horses**: Horses usually receive this medication orally twice daily as tablets ground up and added to feed, or as a special liquid or paste made by your pharmacist.

What Other Information Is Important About This Medication?

- Pentoxifylline should be stored in a tight, light resistant, childproof container away from all children and other household pets.

VETERINARY DRUG HANDBOOK-Client Information Edition
Permission to photocopy for individual clients granted by Gigi Davidson and Donald C. Plumb © 2003

Pergolide

Permax® is another name for this medication.

How Is This Medication Useful?

- Pergolide is used to control the signs and symptoms of Cushing's disease in horses. Horses with Cushing's do not make enough of the brain chemical dopamine. Dopamine controls the secretion of hormones from the pituitary gland, when dopamine is absent, the pituitary gland secretes too many hormones causing diabetes, lameness, and disruptions in the immune system. Pergolide acts like dopamine in the body.

Are There Conditions or Times When Its Use Might Cause More Harm Than Good?

- Pergolide comes from the plant family known as ergot alkaloids. It should not be used in patients who are known to be allergic to these types of plants.
- Pergolide can cause a significant drop in blood pressure when first starting out. It may make your horse "faint". You should know exactly how pergolide is going to affect your horse before using your horse for work or in a performance.
- It is not known whether pergolide is safe to use in pregnancy. It has been used in several pregnant mares without adverse effect, but some mares have also lost foals while taking pergolide. Foals born to mares taking pergolide will need a nurse mare, however, as pergolide will prevent milk letdown in the mare at foaling.
- The tranquilizing drug acepromazine (Promace®) will stop pergolide from acting like dopamine. Acepromazine should not be used regularly in horses on pergolide.
- Pergolide is removed from the body by the liver and kidneys and should be used very carefully in animals with liver or kidney failure.
- If your animal has any of the above conditions, talk to your veterinarian about the potential risks of using the medication versus the benefits that it might have.

What Side Effects Can Be Seen With Its Use?

- The most commonly reported side effect in horses is decrease in or loss of appetite. This effect can be reduced by giving a lower dose.
- Pergolide may also cause stomach and intestinal upset and may cause symptoms of colic in your horse. You should contact your veterinarian immediately if you think your horse is colicking.
- Pergolide can cause a fast or irregular heartbeat.

- Pergolide in high doses can also cause horses to become agitated and unpredictable. Lowering the dose should help resolve this adverse effect. Some humans experience hallucinations while on pergolide and this may be why horses sometimes act "crazy" while taking this drug.
- Pergolide has also caused uncontrolled twitching of the tongue, facial muscles and head.
- When decreasing the dose, it must be done gradually as dropping the dose rapidly can cause hallucinations and behavior changes.

How Should It Be Given?

- Pergolide should be given orally to your horse once daily. It may be given as the tablets for humans, or your pharmacist may compound a flavored liquid or paste for your horse.
- The successful outcome of your animal's treatment with this medication depends upon your commitment and ability to administer it exactly as the veterinarian has prescribed. Please do not skip doses or stop giving the medication. If you have difficulty giving doses consult your veterinarian or pharmacist who can offer administration techniques or change the dosage form to a type of medication that may be more acceptable to you and your animal.
- If you miss a dose of this medication you should give it as soon as you remember it, but if it is within a few hours of the regularly scheduled dose, wait and give it at the regular time. Do not double a dose as this can be toxic to your pet.
- Some other drugs can interact with this medication so tell your veterinarian about any drugs or foods that you currently give your animal. Do not give new foods or medications without first asking your veterinarian.
- **Horses**: Horses usually receive pergolide in doses from 0.25mg to 3mg per horse orally once daily. The horse will be on this medication for the rest of its life as the tumor causing problems in the pituitary is very difficult to remove with surgery and will not go away by itself.

What Other Information Is Important About This Medication?

- Pergolide should be stored in a tight, light resistant, childproof container away from all children and other household pets. It should never be stored at temperatures higher than 86° F, so you should keep it indoors during the hot parts of summer or in climates where the temperature exceeds 86°F. The barn is generally not a good place to store drugs.

Phenobarbital

Luminal®, Solfoton® and phenobarbitone are other names for this medication.

How Is This Medication Useful?

- Phenobarbital is used to control seizures in animals with epilepsy. Because it also causes drowsiness, it has sometimes been used as a tranquilizer/sedative in animals.

Are There Conditions or Times When Its Use Might Cause More Harm Than Good?

- Phenobarbital should not be used in animals that are allergic to it or to drugs like it.
- Phenobarbital is removed from the body by the liver and should be used with extreme caution in animals with liver disease. Phenobarbital may also cause liver disease at higher doses.
- Phenobarbital decreases the ability of the lungs to function properly. It should be used very carefully in animals who have lung disease or lung conditions. Dogs and cats use panting from the lungs to cool themselves, as they cannot sweat. Depressing breathing can not only cause oxygen shortage, but also can cause animals to overheat.
- Phenobarbital has effects on many laboratory tests. Your veterinarian may want to take your animal off phenobarbital prior to doing some tests. You should always remind your veterinarian that your pet is on phenobarbital before performing laboratory tests.
- If your animal has any of the above conditions, talk to your veterinarian about the potential risks of using the medication versus the benefits that it might have.

What Side Effects Can Be Seen With Its Use?

- Phenobarbital most commonly causes tiredness at the beginning of treatment. Some animals will also experience agitation and anxiety at the beginning or treatment. Call your veterinarian if these side effects do not appear to be getting better with time.
- Many animals will eat more, drink more and urinate more when taking phenobarbital.
- Phenobarbital may cause liver damage in higher doses and the dose must be reduced or phenobarbital stopped completely. This is more common in dogs and not very common in cats.
- Phenobarbital also stimulates the production of certain liver enzymes that may indicate the beginning of liver failure. Your veterinarian will want to monitor your pet very closely while on phenobarbital to make sure than none of these side effects are happening.
- Phenobarbital has also rarely suppressed the bone marrow and caused anemias.

How Should It Be Given?

- Phenobarbital may be given by injection at your veterinary clinic or orally at home as a tablet, capsule, liquid, paste or chewable treat. If your cat is extremely difficult to medicate, your veterinarian may prescribe a special topical gel of phenobarbital that can be rubbed into the ears to get into the bloodstream. If you use this topical gel, you must wear gloves while applying and wash hands afterwards. If your job requires you to take random drug tests, you may want to have someone else apply the phenobarbital gel as it may also get into your bloodstream and cause you to fail your blood test. It is usually given twice daily and must be given for the rest of the animal's life or seizures may return.
- The successful outcome of your animal's treatment with this medication depends upon your commitment and ability to administer it exactly as the veterinarian has prescribed. Please do not skip doses or stop giving the medication. If you have difficulty giving doses consult your veterinarian or pharmacist who can offer administration techniques or change the dosage form to a type of medication that may be more acceptable to you and your animal.
- If you miss a dose of this medication you should give it as soon as you remember it, but if it is within a few hours of the regularly scheduled dose, wait and give it at the regular time. Do not double a dose as this can be toxic to your pet.
- Some other drugs can interact with this medication so tell your veterinarian about any drugs or foods that you currently give your animal. Do not give new foods or medications without first asking your veterinarian.
- **Dogs and Cats**: Dogs and cats usually receive phenobarbital orally once or twice daily. It must be given for life to control epilepsy.
- **Horses**: Horses with seizures can be very dangerous to themselves and others. Phenobarbital is rarely used for long term in horses, but when used is given once daily. It is considered a Class 2 Drug by the Association of Racing Commissioners International (ARCI).

What Other Information Is Important About This Medication?

- Phenobarbital should be stored in a tight, light resistant, childproof container away from all children and other household pets.
- Phenobarbital is a Schedule IV controlled substance. You will need to get a new prescription from your veterinarian once every 6 months.

Phenoxybenzamine

Dibenzyline® is another name for this medication.

How Is This Medication Useful?

- Phenoxybenzamine is a drug used to relax the bladder and urethra muscles during bladder and urethral spasms that are causing urine to leak out of the body.
- It is also used to reduce the blood pressure in animals suffering from a tumor known as pheochromocytoma.
- It has been used in horses to treat or prevent lameness (laminitis) and to treat diarrhea in horses.

Are There Conditions or Times When Its Use Might Cause More Harm Than Good?

- Phenoxybenzamine should not be used in horses with signs of colic.
- Pets suffering from shock or very low blood pressure should not receive phenoxybenzamine.
- Phenoxybenzamine can cause a rapid heartbeat and should be used very carefully if at all in animals with heart disease.
- Phenoxybenzamine may cause failure to ejaculate and should be used with caution in males intended for breeding.
- Phenoxybenzamine should be used carefully in animals with kidney disease.
- If your animal has any of the above conditions, talk to your veterinarian about the potential risks of using the medication versus the benefits that it might have.

What Side Effects Can Be Seen With Its Use?

- Phenoxybenzamine can cause a significant drop in blood pressure. If your animal appears to faint or is excessively tired and weak or dizzy, you should contact your veterinarian immediately.
- Phenoxybenzamine can cause stomach upset and vomiting. It may cause constipation in horses and may lead to colic.
- Phenoxybenazmine has also caused a stuffy or runny nose, pinpoint pupils of the eye, fast heart beat and failure to ejaculate.

How Should It Be Given?

- Phenoxybenzamine is not available as a commercial drug. You will need to contact a compounding pharmacist to obtain phenoxybenzamine. It may be compounded into capsules, chewable treats, or liquid dosage forms. It is usually given from once to three times daily.

- The successful outcome of your animal's treatment with this medication depends upon your commitment and ability to administer it exactly as the veterinarian has prescribed. Please do not skip doses or stop giving the medication. If you have difficulty giving doses consult your veterinarian or pharmacist who can offer administration techniques or change the dosage form to a type of medication that may be more acceptable to you and your animal.
- If you miss a dose of this medication you should give it as soon as you remember it, but if it is within a few hours of the regularly scheduled dose, wait and give it at the regular time. Do not double a dose as this can be toxic to your pet.
- Some other drugs can interact with this medication so tell your veterinarian about any drugs or foods that you currently give your animal. Do not give new foods or medications without first asking your veterinarian.
- **Dogs and Cats**: Phenoxybenzamine is usually given orally once or twice daily with food.
- **Horses**: Phenoxybenzamine is usually given by injection for lameness in horses. It can be given orally up to twice daily for diarrhea. When used in horses, it is considered a Class 3 drug by the Association of Racing Commissioners International (ARCI).

What Other Information Is Important About This Medication?

- Phenoxybenzamine should be stored in a tight, light resistant, childproof container away from all children and other household pets.
- As phenoxybenzamine must be compounded by a pharmacist, you should call for refills a few days ahead of time to allow for preparation of the drug.

Phenylbutazone

Butazolidin®, Phenylzone®, Butatab®, Phenylbute® and bute are other names for this medication.

How Is This Medication Useful?

- Phenylbutazone is a non-steroidal antiinflammatory drug used to treat pain and inflammation in horses.

Are There Conditions or Times When Its Use Might Cause More Harm Than Good?

- Phenylbutazone should not be used in animals that are allergic or are allergic to other antiinflammatory drugs like it.
- Phenylbutazone should not be given to animals that are going to be used for human food.
- If given in an artery, phenylbutazone can cause seizures in the horse. When injected, it should only be given into the veins and not injected into the muscle or under the skin. It is very very painful when injected into the muscle and will cause muscle damage.
- Phenylbutazone can inhibit the enzymes that protect the stomach, kidneys and blood cells. It should not be used in animals that have or have a history of stomach ulcers. The drug misoprostol may be given at the same time as phenylbutazone to help prevent these stomach side effects.
- Phenylbutazone can stop the bone marrow from producing blood cells. It should not be used in animals that are anemic or have bleeding disorders.
- Phenylbutazone can damage the kidneys and should not be used in animals that have kidney disease and should not be used in combination with other drugs that may cause kidney disease. You should leave out plenty of fresh water for your horses while on this medication as lack of adequate water intake will worsen the effects of this drug on the kidneys.
- Phenylbutazone may mask the signs of lameness and it is unethical to use it in horses prior to soundness exams.
- Phenylbutazone may be particularly toxic to foals and ponies and probably should not be used in these animals.
- Phenylbutazone should probably not be used in pregnant mares as it has been shown to cause birth defects in laboratory animals.

- Phenylbutazone can alter the results of laboratory tests. You should let your veterinarian know if your horse is on phenylbutazone prior to having any laboratory tests performed.
- If your animal has any of the above conditions, talk to your veterinarian about the potential risks of using the medication versus the benefits that it might have.

What Side Effects Can Be Seen With Its Use?

- Phenylbutazone can cause stomach upset and vomiting. It may irritate the stomach to the point of ulcers in the mouth and stomach. If your horse acts like it is in pain or grinds its teeth, you should contact your veterinarian immediately.
- Phenylbutazone can cause kidney damage. If your horse changes its drinking or urinating habits you should contact your veterinarian immediately.
- Phenylbutazone may cause a loss of appetite. If your horse stops eating your should contact your veterinarian.

How Should It Be Given?

- Phenylbutazone may be given to your horse as an injection into the vein. It should only be given into the veins and not injected into the arteries, muscle or under the skin. It is very painful when injected into the muscle and will cause muscle damage. Injectable phenylbutazone should be stored in the refrigerator and protected from light.
- Phenylbutazone is most often given to your horse as an oral powder, paste or tablet. You should give it with food.
- The successful outcome of your animal's treatment with this medication depends upon your commitment and ability to administer it exactly as the veterinarian has prescribed. Please do not skip doses or stop giving the medication. If you have difficulty giving doses consult your veterinarian or pharmacist who can offer administration techniques or change the dosage form to a type of medication that may be more acceptable to you and your animal.

(Continued on following page)

VETERINARY DRUG HANDBOOK-Client Information Edition
Permission to photocopy for individual clients granted by Gigi Davidson and Donald C. Plumb © 2003

Phenylbutazone

How Should It Be Given? (continued from previous page)

- If you miss a dose of this medication you should give it as soon as you remember it, but if it is within a few hours of the regularly scheduled dose, wait and give it at the regular time. Do not double a dose as this can be toxic to your horse.
- Some other drugs can interact with this medication so tell your veterinarian about any drugs or foods that you currently give your animal. Do not give new foods or medications without first asking your veterinarian.
- **Dogs and Cats**: Phenylbutazone is rarely used in dogs as it is more toxic than the newer anti-inflammatory agents such as Rimadyl®, Etogesic® and Deramaxx®. It is generally not used in cats.
- **Horses**: Horses usually receive phenylbutazone as an oral paste or tablet once or twice daily with food. If injected, it should only be injected in the vein and not in the arteries, muscle or under the skin as it will cause serious adverse effects such as seizures and pain if given by these routes.

What Other Information Is Important About This Medication?

- Phenylbutazone should be stored in a tight, light resistant, childproof container away from all children and other household pets. Phenylbutazone injection should be stored in the refrigerator protected from light.
- Phenylbutazone injection should not be mixed with other drugs in the same syringe.

Phenylpropanolamine

Proin® and Propadrine® are other names for this medication.

How Is This Medication Useful?

- Phenylpropanolamine is used to tighten up the bladder sphincter for animals suffering from urine leakage (incontinence).
- Phenylpropanolamine was taken off the human market in 1999 because it caused extreme high blood pressure and some strokes in some humans. It has not been reported to cause these effects in animals when used at normal doses.

Are There Conditions or Times When Its Use Might Cause More Harm Than Good?

- Phenylpropanolamine should not be used in animals with glaucoma, prostate disease, overactive thyroid, diabetes, heart disease or high blood pressure.
- Phenylpropanolamine should not be used within 2 weeks of drugs known as MAO inhibitors (Mitaban® Dip, Preventic® Flea Collars, Anipryl®, and isoniazid are a few of these drugs). When phenylpropanolamine is given with these drugs it can cause serious increases in blood pressure that can cause death. Aged cheese can also cause this effect, so make sure that your pets do not get into any aged cheese while on this drug. If your pet is receiving any of these medications, your veterinarian will ask you to stop giving them for at least 2-5 weeks before he prescribes phenylpropanolamine.
- Phenylpropanolamine should not be used in pregnant or nursing animals.
- Phenylpropanolamine may cause an irregular heartbeat if used in combination with a drug called digoxin.
- If your animal has any of the above conditions, talk to your veterinarian about the potential risks of using the medication versus the benefits that it might have.

What Side Effects Can Be Seen With Its Use?

- Phenylpropanolamine is a stimulant that may cause restlessness, irritability, high blood pressure and loss of appetite. It may also cause a rapid heart beat.
- If your pet shows any of these signs you should consult your veterinarian for advice.

How Should It Be Given?

- Phenylpropanolamine should be given once or twice daily orally. It should be given at bedtime to be sure that the drug lasts all through the night and the pet does not have accidents in the middle of the night.
- Phenylpropanolamine is available as a chewable treat, an oral liquid or a longer acting capsule. It is extremely bitter, so you may want to hide it in some food.
- The successful outcome of your animal's treatment with this medication depends upon your commitment and ability to administer it exactly as the veterinarian has prescribed. Please do not skip doses or stop giving the medication. If you have difficulty giving doses consult your veterinarian or pharmacist who can offer administration techniques or change the dosage form to a type of medication that may be more acceptable to you and your animal.
- If you miss a dose of this medication you should give it as soon as you remember it, but if it is within a few hours of the regularly scheduled dose, wait and give it at the regular time. Do not double a dose as this can be toxic to your pet.
- Some other drugs can interact with this medication so tell your veterinarian about any drugs or foods that you currently give your animal. Do not give new foods or medications without first asking your veterinarian.
- **Dogs and Cats**: Dogs and cats usually receive phenylpropanolamine orally once or twice daily. It should be given as late in the evening as possible (bedtime) to prevent accidents during the night. Do not give your pet aged cheese or use tick collars while on this medication.

What Other Information Is Important About This Medication?

- Phenylpropanolamine should be stored in a tight, light resistant, childproof container away from all children and other household pets.
- Phenylpropanolamine has been banned by the FDA for use in humans.
- Phenylpropanolamine is not used is horses and is considered a Class 3 drug by the Association of Racing Commissioners International (ARCI).

Phytonadione (Vitamin K₁)

K-Caps®, Veda-K1®, Veta-K1® and Mephyton® are other names for this medication.

How Is This Medication Useful?

- Phytonadione or Vitamin K1 is used by the body to produce factors in the blood to help it coagulate and prevent bleeding. It is often used after animals eat mouse or rat poisons (anticoagulant rodenticides) that can cause severe bleeding. Because some of these poisons can stay in the body for a long time, treatment with phytonadione may be required for several weeks.

Are There Conditions or Times When Its Use Might Cause More Harm Than Good?

- When given by mouth for anticoagulant rodenticide poisoning, phytonadione is considered very safe.
- Phytonadione is not considered to be useful for treating bleeding caused by liver problems.
- While not proven to be safe to use during pregnancy, potential benefits to the mother and offspring generally far outweigh any risks.

What Side Effects Can Be Seen With Its Use?

- When given by mouth (orally), side effects caused by phytonadione are very unlikely.
- If given by injection by your veterinarian, bleeding at the site of injection can occur.
- If given into the vein (intravenously), life-threatening allergic reactions can occur and this method of giving the drug is not usually recommended.

How Should It Be Given?

- Depending on the severity of the poisoning, your veterinarian may prescribe the drug to be given once to three times a day for several weeks. It is very important that all doses are given even if the animal appears to be fine, or bleeding can again start.
- If you miss a dose, give it as soon as you remember. If it is now time for the next dose, give both doses at that time.
- To improve the drug's absorption form the gastrointestinal tract, it is best to give the medication with food that has a high fat content. Your veterinarian can advise you on your animal's diet during therapy.

- The successful outcome of your animal's treatment with this medication depends upon your commitment and ability to administer it exactly as the veterinarian has prescribed. Please do not skip doses or stop giving the medication. If you have difficulty giving doses consult your veterinarian or pharmacist who can offer administration techniques or change the dosage form to a type of medication that may be more acceptable to you and your animal.
- If you miss a dose of this medication you should give it as soon as you remember it, but if it is within a few hours of the regularly scheduled dose, wait and give it at the regular time. Do not double a dose as this can be toxic to your pet.
- Some other drugs can interact with this medication so tell your veterinarian about any drugs or foods that you currently give your animal. Do not give new foods or medications without first asking your veterinarian.
- **Dogs and Cats**: Dogs and cats usually receive vitamin K as an oral capsule once or twice daily for several weeks. If your pet needs a very small dose, your veterinarian may ask you to give the injectable form of vitamin K by mouth. It is very bitter, so your pharmacist may be able to flavor the injection so that it will be more acceptable to your pet.

What Other Information Is Important About This Medication?

- Your veterinarian may advise you to keep your animal quiet during therapy to reduce the chance of bleeding occurring.
- Store the capsules and tablets in a light-resistant container at room temperature.
- If you have any other questions about this drug, be sure to ask your veterinarian or pharmacist.

Piperazine

Pipa-Tabs® is another name for this medication. There are many "wormer" products for dogs and cats that are available without a prescription that contain piperazine. Several of these are from Sergent's or Hart's Mountain.

How Is This Medication Useful?

- Piperazine is an orally administered drug that kills roundworms (ascarids) in the gastrointestinal tract in a variety of species, including dogs and cats.

Are There Conditions or Times When Its Use Might Cause More Harm Than Good?

- Piperazine should not be used in animals with chronic liver or kidney disease or in animals who have digestive problems such as chronic constipation.
- Piperazine should be used cautiously in dogs or cats that have seizures (epilepsy).
- Rupture or blockage of intestines is possible in horses who have heavy infestations of roundworms.
- Piperazine is not effective against many types of gastrointestinal parasites and should not be used for parasites other than ascarids.

What Side Effects Can Be Seen With Its Use?

- In dogs or cats, adverse effects with piperazine are uncommon when given at recommended dosages, but diarrhea, vomiting and unsteadiness (ataxia) may be seen.
- In horses or foals, adverse effects with piperazine are uncommon when given at recommended dosages, but soft feces may be seen.
- Because overdoses of piperazine may cause serious effects be sure to give the drug as instructed.
- Side effects of overdoses in cats or dogs can include vomiting, weakness, difficulty breathing, muscle twitches, rear leg unsteadiness, increased salivation, depression, dehydration, head-pressing, and eye and pupil changes. If these occur, contact your veterinarian.

How Should It Be Given?

- The successful outcome of your animal's treatment with this medication depends upon your commitment and ability to administer it exactly as the veterinarian has prescribed. Please do not skip doses or stop giving the medication. If you have difficulty giving doses consult your veterinarian or pharmacist who can offer administration techniques or change the dosage form to a type of medication that may be more acceptable to you and your animal
- Because some other drugs can interact with this medication, you should tell your veterinarian about any drugs or foods that you currently give your animal. Do not give new foods or medications without first asking your veterinarian.
- **Dogs and Cats:** The medication is usually given by mouth one time and then repeated in a few weeks.

What Other Information Is Important About This Medication?

- Do not use laxatives or purgatives with piperazine as they may cause the drug to be eliminated form the body before it is fully effective.
- Do not give with other "wormers" unless instructed to do so by your veterinarian.
- If you have any other questions about this drug, be sure to ask your veterinarian or pharmacist

VETERINARY DRUG HANDBOOK-Client Information Edition
Permission to photocopy for individual clients granted by Gigi Davidson and Donald C. Plumb © 2003

Piroxicam

Feldene® is another name for this medication.

How Is This Medication Useful?

- Piroxicam's primary use in dogs and cats has been as a supplementary drug to use in the treatment of certain types of cancers, especially those found in the bladder. Piroxicam probably acts by enhancing the body's own ability to destroy cancer cells. Piroxicam is in the non-steroidal anti-inflammatory (NSAID) class of drugs and is commonly used in people for treating arthritic symptoms. While it can be used for this purpose in dogs, there are safer drugs to use.

Are There Conditions or Times When Its Use Might Cause More Harm Than Good?

- Piroxicam should not be used in animals who are allergic to it or severely allergic to other drugs like it (such as aspirin).
- Use this drug very cautiously, if at all, in animals that have active stomach or gastrointestinal ulcers or have had these kinds of ulcers in the past. Piroxicam can make these ulcers worse or reappear.
- If your animal has severe heart disease, talk to your veterinarian about the risks of piroxicam making edema (swelling) worse.
- Piroxicam must be used in cats very cautiously; there is little experience using this drug in this species and cats often do not tolerate these class of drugs well.

What Side Effects Can Be Seen With Its Use?

- The most commonly reported side effects in animals taking piroxicam are usually related to it causing stomach bleeding and ulcers. This may present as decreased appetite, vomiting (including blood in the vomit), diarrhea, or blood in the stools. If you see "tarry" black stools contact your veterinarian. If stomach ulcers occur, your veterinarian may prescribe other medicines to help control them.
- Piroxicam may also affect the kidneys or the liver. Tell your veterinarian if your animal's urinary habits have changed while receiving this drug.
- Piroxicam may cause your animal to bleed longer after cuts than usual. This is usually not a serious problem, but contact your veterinarian if you note anything unusual.

How Should It Be Given?

- The successful outcome of your animal's treatment with this medication depends upon your commitment and ability to administer it exactly as the veterinarian has prescribed. Please do not skip doses or stop giving the medication. If you have difficulty giving doses consult your veterinarian or pharmacist who can offer administration techniques or change the dosage form to a type of medication that may be more acceptable to you and your animal.
- Some other drugs can interact with this medication so tell your veterinarian about any drugs or foods that you currently give your animal. Do not give new foods or medications without first asking your veterinarian.
- **Dogs**: Dogs usually receive this medication once a day by mouth.
- Try to give this medication with food as that may reduce the chances of stomach problems occurring.
- If you miss a dose of this medication you should give it as soon as you remember it if it is within 12 hours of when you should have given it. Otherwise skip this dose and give the next dose at the regular time. Do not double a dose as this can be toxic to your dog.

What Other Information Is Important About This Medication?

- Keep the capsules stored in the original prescription vial at room temperature; do not expose them to high heat.
- Because of the differences in size between animals and people, your veterinarian may compound or have compounded by a pharmacy capsule strengths that are smaller than are originally manufactured.

Praziquantel

Droncit®, Drontal®, Drontal Plus®, Cutter Tape Tabs®
are other names for this medication.

How Is This Medication Useful?

• Praziquantel is used to kill intestinal tapeworms
  and some other types of parasites.

Are There Conditions or Times When Its Use Might Cause More Harm Than Good?

• Praziquantel should not be used in puppies less
  than 4 weeks old and kittens less than 6 weeks
  old unless indicated on the product labeling or
  authorized by your veterinarian.
• Praziquantel is considered safe for use in pregnant animals.
• If your animal has any of the above conditions,
  talk to your veterinarian about the potential
  risks of using the medication versus the benefits
  that it might have.

What Side Effects Can Be Seen With Its Use?

• Side effects are rare, but praziquantel can cause
  loss of appetite, diarrhea, vomiting and drooling.
• The injection can cause pain at the injection site.
• Some cats will show signs of weakness and staggering after praziquantel administration.
• If your pet shows any of the above signs, you
  should contact your veterinarian immediately.
• If your animal has a large load of tapeworms,
  they may be expelled in the feces. Usually, however the tapeworms are digested before they
  come out in the feces.

How Should It Be Given?

• Praziquantel is given with or without food as a
  single dose. If your pet is large, your veterinarian
  may give you several tablets to give at one time.
  Make sure that your pet swallows all of the
  medication. Your veterinarian may ask you to
  repeat a dose in a few weeks to make sure that
  all forms of the parasite are dead.

• The successful outcome of your animal's treatment with this medication depends upon your
  commitment and ability to administer it exactly
  as the veterinarian has prescribed. Please do not
  skip doses or stop giving the medication. If you
  have difficulty giving doses consult your veterinarian or pharmacist who can offer administration techniques or change the dosage form to a
  type of medication that may be more acceptable
  to you and your animal.
• Some other drugs can interact with this medication so tell your veterinarian about any drugs or
  foods that you currently give your animal. Do
  not give new foods or medications without first
  asking your veterinarian.
• **Dogs and Cats**: Dogs and cats usually receive
  this medication orally as a single dose. Your veterinarian may ask you to give the tablets once
  more in 2-3 weeks to ensure that all the parasites are dead.
• **Birds and Reptiles**: Birds and reptiles may receive this medication orally and the dose is repeated in 2 weeks. Often your veterinarian will
  give this drug by injection at the clinic to reptiles
  and birds.

What Other Information Is Important About This Medication?

• Praziquantel should be stored in a tight, light
  resistant, childproof container away from all
  children and other household pets.

VETERINARY DRUG HANDBOOK-Client Information Edition
Permission to photocopy for individual clients granted by Gigi Davidson and Donald C. Plumb © 2003

Prednisone
Prednisolone

Prednis-tab®, Cortef®, Prelone®, Solu-Delta-Cortef® are other names for this medication.

How Is This Medication Useful?

- Prednisone and prednisolone are glucocorticoid drugs (like the hormone cortisol) used for many indications. They affect nearly every cell in the body and can be used to suppress the immune system in diseases like lupus, to stop itching, to treat Addison's Disease, to treat certain types of cancer, to stop swelling of the brain, to treat certain kinds of anemia and many other diseases and conditions. You should ask your veterinarian specifically why this medication is being used in your pet.

Are There Conditions or Times When Its Use Might Cause More Harm Than Good?

- Prednisone and drugs like it should not be used in patients that have a fungus infection, as this will cause significant worsening of the fungal condition.
- Some kinds of mange are worsened with the use of prednisone and drugs like it.
- Prednisone and drugs like it should always be given with food to prevent stomach ulcers and bleeding that are sometimes associated with oral corticosteroid therapy.
- Animals with Cushing's disease are already making too much cortisol and should only receive glucocorticoid drugs during stressful events or when your veterinarian recommends them.
- Prednisone and other glucocorticoids may stunt the growth of developing animals and should be used with extreme caution in young animals.
- Predisone and drugs like it significantly alter the effect of other medications. You should not give it at the same time as other anti-flammatory drugs (NSAIDs) such as aspirin or carprofen (Rimadyl®, Etogesic®, or Deramaxx®). You should always tell you veterinarian about any other medications that you are giving your pet.
- Glucocorticoids also affect the results of many laboratory tests. You should always tell your veterinarian about any medications that you are giving your pet prior to a laboratory test of any kind.
- Prednisone must be converted to the active form of the drug, prednisolone, in the liver. If your pet has liver disease, then your veterinarian will probably prescribe prednisolone instead of prednisone.

- Prednisone does not work as well orally in horses as prednisolone does , and your veterinarian will probably prescribe prednisolone if your horse needs a glucocorticoid.
- If your pet has been on high doses of prednisone or other immunosuppressive drugs, you should not have it vaccinated without your veterinarian's advice as the vaccine may not work or may actually give your pet the disease that you are trying to prevent.
- Animals who have received prednisone and drugs like it for a long time should not be taken off the drug suddenly as their bodies may not return to making their own cortisol hormone. Cortisol and prednisone help your pet handle stressful events so you should ask your veterinarian before stopping any prednisone therapy.
- Prednisone and drugs like it should be used very carefully in diabetic pets as these drugs will alter blood sugar and the amount of insulin that your pet needs.
- Prednisone therapy may cause your horse to go into early labor if administered during the later parts of pregnancy.
- If your animal has any of the above conditions, talk to your veterinarian about the potential risks of using the medication versus the benefits that it might have.

What Side Effects Can Be Seen With Its Use?

- Animals treated with prednisone will have an increased appetite, increased thirst and an increased need to urinate. You should be aware that your pet may need to go out more frequently to urinate. As it is stressful to some pets to have "accidents" you should make sure that your pet can go outside or have a clean litter box when needed.
- Glucocorticoid drugs will suppress your animal's immune system and may increase the risk for infection. If your pet shows any signs of fever (103-105°F in most dogs and cats), or acts like it has a urinary tract infection (frequent or painful urination) you should contact your veterinarian immediately.

(Continued on following page)

Prednisone
Prednisolone
(continued)

What Side Effects Can Be Seen With Its Use? (continued from previous page)

- Some animals on long-term therapy with prednisone will develop Cushing's disease. If your pet shows signs of dry hair coat or hair loss, weakness and muscle loss, darkening of the skin, or develops a pot-belly, you should contact your veterinarian.
- Some animals may become aggressive while on prednisone. You should contact your veterinarian if this behavior change occurs or does not go away with time.
- Prednisone will cause changes in your pet's insulin requirements if it is a diabetic. You should ask your veterinarian for instructions on how to deal with these changes if your pet is receiving insulin injections.

How Should It Be Given?

- Prednisone and other glucocorticoid drugs should be given orally with food to reduce the chances of stomach ulcers or irritation. If given once daily, prednisone is usually given in the morning to dogs and horses, and in the evening to cats as this will more closely mimic their natural hormone cycles.
- The successful outcome of your animal's treatment with this medication depends upon your commitment and ability to administer it exactly as the veterinarian has prescribed. Please do not skip doses or stop giving the medication. If you have difficulty giving doses consult your veterinarian or pharmacist who can offer administration techniques or change the dosage form to a type of medication that may be more acceptable to you and your animal.
- If you miss a dose of this medication you should give it as soon as you remember it, but if it is within a few hours of the regularly scheduled dose, wait and give it at the regular time. Do not double a dose as this can be toxic to your pet.

- Some other drugs can interact with this medication so tell your veterinarian about any drugs or foods that you currently give your animal. Do not give new foods or medications without first asking your veterinarian.
- **Dogs and Cats**: Dogs and cats usually receive prednisone and prednisolone orally once to twice daily. Dogs usually receive prednisone in the morning and cats usually receive it in the evening if only given once daily as this will more closely mimic their natural hormone cycles. Commercially available prednisone liquids are very repulsive to cats. Your pharmacist may compound a specially flavored oral liquid of prednisone or prednisolone to increase your cat's acceptance of the medication.
- **Horses**: Horses generally do not receive long term glucocorticoid therapy, but if they do, they receive it orally once daily mixed in the feed. Prednisolone is a better choice than prednisone when given orally to horses. Prednisolone and prednisone are considered Class 4 drugs by the Association of Racing Commissioners International (ARCI).

What Other Information Is Important About This Medication?

- Prednisone and prednisolone should be stored at room temperature in a tight, light resistant, childproof container away from all children and other household pets.

Propantheline Bromide

Probanthine® is another name for this medication.

How Is This Medication Useful?

- Propantheline is a drug that acts on smooth muscles and is used to treat urine leaking, certain diarrheas, heart disorders, and to relax the rectum for rectal examination in horses.

Are There Conditions or Times When Its Use Might Cause More Harm Than Good?

- Propantheline should not be used in patients who have shown an allergy to it or a sensitivity to other agents like it (anticholinergics agents). Tell your veterinarian if your pet has ever had a reaction to a drug or did not tolerate the effects of a drug.
- It should probably not be used in animals with a rapid heartbeat due to heart disease or an overactive thyroid.
- Propantheline should not be used in animals that have a stomach or an intestinal blockage or stoppage.
- Propantheline should not be used in patients with myasthenia gravis except as an antidote for an overdose of the drugs (usually pyridostigmine) used to treat myasthenia gravis.
- Propantheline is removed from the body by the liver and the kidneys and should be used carefully in animals with liver or kidney disease.
- If your animal has any of the above conditions, talk to your veterinarian about the potential risks of using the medication versus the benefits that it might have.

What Side Effects Can Be Seen With Its Use?

- Propantheline can cause dry mouth, dry eyes, inability to urinate, fast heart beat, and constipation. If your pet shows any of these signs you should contact your veterinarian.
- Vomiting and drooling have also been reported in cats.
- Propantheline can also stop the movement of the intestines and may cause overgrowth of the bacteria in the stomach and intestines, leading to bloat and colic.

How Should It Be Given?

- Propantheline should be given orally on an empty stomach as food will keep the drug from getting into the bloodstream. It is usually given orally once to three times daily.
- The successful outcome of your animal's treatment with this medication depends upon your commitment and ability to administer it exactly as the veterinarian has prescribed. Please do not skip doses or stop giving the medication. If you have difficulty giving doses consult your veterinarian or pharmacist who can offer administration techniques or change the dosage form to a type of medication that may be more acceptable to you and your animal.
- If you miss a dose of this medication you should give it as soon as you remember it, but if it is within a few hours of the regularly scheduled dose, wait and give it at the regular time. Do not double a dose as this can be toxic to your pet.
- Some other drugs can interact with this medication so tell your veterinarian about any drugs or foods that you currently give your animal. Do not give new foods or medications without first asking your veterinarian.
- **Dogs and Cats**: Dogs and cats usually receive this medication orally once to three times daily. It should be given on an empty stomach.
- **Horses**: Horses do not usually receive this drug orally because of the risk of colic, but it may be given by injection by your veterinarian to relax the rectum prior to rectal examination, reducing the risk of tearing the rectal wall during examination. Propantheline is considered a Class 4 Drug by the Association of Racing Commissioners International (ARCI).

What Other Information Is Important About This Medication?

- Propanthline should be stored in a tight, light resistant, childproof container away from all children and other household pets.
- Propantheline may have to be compounded by a compounding pharmacist due to limited supplies of commercially available drug.

Permission to photocopy for individual clients granted by Gigi Davidson and Donald C. Plumb © 2003

Propranolol

Inderal® is another name for this medication.

How Is This Medication Useful?

- Propranolol is a drug used to regulate your pet's heartbeat and improve the performance of the heart in certain kinds of disease.

Are There Conditions or Times When Its Use Might Cause More Harm Than Good?

- Propranolol should be used carefully, if at all, in animals with heart failure or a very slow heartbeat.
- Propranolol may cause lung spasm and should be used very carefully, if at all, in patients with asthma or other lung diseases.
- Propranolol is removed from the body by the liver and kidneys and should be used carefully in patients with liver and kidney disease.
- Propranolol can mask the signs of low blood sugar and should be used very carefully in pets with diabetes. If your diabetic pet receives propranolol, your veterinarian should tell you exactly what to watch for to make sure that it is not getting dangerously low blood sugar levels.
- Propranolol may also mask the signs of an overactive thyroid and should be used carefully if at all in patients with hyperthyroidism (overactive thyroid).
- Propranolol should be used carefully in patients who are already being treated with a drug called digoxin as propranolol may cause the digoxin to become toxic in your pet.
- Many drugs will affect or be affected by propranolol. You should tell your veterinarian about any medications that you are giving your pet.
- If your animal has any of the above conditions, talk to your veterinarian about the potential risks of using the medication versus the benefits that it might have.

What Side Effects Can Be Seen With Its Use?

- Propranolol does not have many side effects when used properly. Some animals may develop a very slow heartbeat, become more tired and depressed than usual, and have lower blood pressure than usual.
- Some animals may develop low blood pressure, low blood sugar, diarrhea, and difficulty breathing while receiving propranolol.

How Should It Be Given?

- Propranolol is usually given orally once to three times daily in pets. Oral doses are much higher than injectable or transdermal doses because of the effects of the stomach and liver on getting drugs into the blood.
- The successful outcome of your animal's treatment with this medication depends upon your commitment and ability to administer it exactly as the veterinarian has prescribed. Please do not skip doses or stop giving the medication. If you have difficulty giving doses consult your veterinarian or pharmacist who can offer administration techniques or change the dosage form to a type of medication that may be more acceptable to you and your animal.
- If you miss a dose of this medication you should give it as soon as you remember it, but if it is within a few hours of the regularly scheduled dose, wait and give it at the regular time. Do not double a dose as this can be toxic to your pet.
- Some other drugs can interact with this medication so tell your veterinarian about any drugs or foods that you currently give your animal. Do not give new foods or medications without first asking your veterinarian.
- **Dogs and Cats**: Dogs and cats usually receive propranolol orally once to three times daily.
- **Horses**: Horses don't usually receive propranolol, but may get it orally three times daily. Because of the effects on blood pressure, a lower dose is usually started on horses and increased as the horse begins to tolerate the side effects of the medication. Propranolol is considered a Class 3 Drug by the Association of Racing Commissioners International (ARCI).

What Other Information Is Important About This Medication?

- Propranolol should be stored in a tight, light resistant, childproof container away from all children and other household pets.

VETERINARY DRUG HANDBOOK-Client Information Edition
Permission to photocopy for individual clients granted by Gigi Davidson and Donald C. Plumb © 2003

Pyrantel Pamoate

Nemex® and Strongid-T®are other names for this medication.

How Is This Medication Useful?

- Pyrantel is an orally administered anthelmintic (wormer) that is effective against a variety of roundworms and hookworms in dogs, cats, horses, birds and rabbits. It is also used to treat pinworms in humans.

Are There Conditions or Times When Its Use Might Cause More Harm Than Good?

- Pyrantel should be used with caution in severely debilitated animals.

What Side Effects Can Be Seen With Its Use?

- Side effects are uncommon with this medication. Occasionally some animals may vomit after receiving it.
- While very safe at usual doses, large overdoses of pyrantel given over a period of time can cause serious effects.

How Should It Be Given?

- Be certain to give this drug exactly as your veterinarian prescribes. Please do not skip doses or stop giving the medication or re-treatment may be necessary. Consult your veterinarian or pharmacist who can offer administration techniques or change the dosage form to a type of medication that may be more acceptable to you and your animal.
- If you miss a dose of this medication you should give it as soon as you remember it. Do not double doses as this will not increase the effectiveness of the treatment.
- Some other drugs can interact with this medication so tell your veterinarian about any drugs or foods that you currently give your animal. Do not give new foods or medications without first asking your veterinarian.
- **Dogs and Cats**: Dogs and cats usually receive this drug orally once and then the dose is repeated at least once every one to three weeks.

What Other Information Is Important About This Medication?

- Pyrantel should be stored at room temperature in a tight, childproof container away from all children and other household pets.
- If using the oral suspension be sure to shake it well before giving.

Pyridostigmine

Mestinon® is another name for this medication.

How Is This Medication Useful?

- Pyridostigmine is a drug called a cholinesterase inhibitor and allows the weakened muscles of pets with myasthenia gravis to work better.

Are There Conditions or Times When Its Use Might Cause More Harm Than Good?

- Pyridostigmine should be used with caution, if at all, in animals with lung spasm, slow or irregular heart beat, stomach ulcers, epilepsy or overactive thyroid.
- Cats are particularly sensitive to cholinesterase inhibitors and pyridostigmine should be used with extreme caution in this species.
- Pyridostigmine should not be used in animals with a bladder or stomach blockage.
- Pyridostigmine should not be used in animals that are allergic to it or to drugs like it.
- Pyridostigmine should be used very carefully in pregnant mothers as it may cause early labor and may also cause muscle weakness in the babies.
- If your animal has any of the above conditions, talk to your veterinarian about the potential risks of using the medication versus the benefits that it might have.

What Side Effects Can Be Seen With Its Use?

- Known side effects of pyridostigmine include vomiting, diarrhea, drooling, lung spasm, pinpoint pupils, blurry vision, watery eyes, irregular (too fast or too slow) heart beat, heart spasm, low blood pressure, muscle spasm and weakness.
- If your pet shows any signs of these adverse effects, you should call your veterinarian.

How Should It Be Given?

- Pyridostigmine may be given as oral tablets or liquid, but you should not switch your pet back and forth between tablets and liquid because this can change the amount of drug that gets into your pet's bloodstream.

- The successful outcome of your animal's treatment with this medication depends upon your commitment and ability to administer it exactly as the veterinarian has prescribed. Please do not skip doses or stop giving the medication. If you have difficulty giving doses consult your veterinarian or pharmacist who can offer administration techniques or change the dosage form to a type of medication that may be more acceptable to you and your animal.
- If you miss a dose of this medication you should give it as soon as you remember it, but if it is within a few hours of the regularly scheduled dose, wait and give it at the regular time. Do not double a dose as this can be toxic to your pet.
- Some other drugs can interact with this medication so tell your veterinarian about any drugs or foods that you currently give your animal. Do not give new foods or medications without first asking your veterinarian.
- **Dogs and Cats**: Dogs usually receive pyridostigmine orally two to three times daily. Cats rarely receive this drug, but if they do, it is given only once daily.
- **Horses**: Horses do not usually receive this drug.

What Other Information Is Important About This Medication?

- Pyridostigmine should be stored in a tight, light resistant, childproof container away from all children and other household pets.
- Other liquid drugs containing an ingredient called methylcellulose should not be given at the same time as pyridostigmine as it can inactivate the drug.
- Please give medication exactly the way your veterinarian prescribes and do not switch administered forms of the drug without your veterinarian's advice (e.g.: do not switch from tablets to liquid or from commercially available liquid to specially compounded liquid) as this may alter the effect of the drug and cause your pet to come out of remission.
- You should elevate the food bowl while feeding your pet to avoid any risk of aspiration (inhaling food into the lungs) due to weak swallowing muscles.

VETERINARY DRUG HANDBOOK-Client Information Edition
Permission to photocopy for individual clients granted by Gigi Davidson and Donald C. Plumb © 2003

Ranitidine

Zantac® is another name for this medication.

How Is This Medication Useful?

- Ranitidine is used to decrease acid secretion in the stomach and protect against the formation of ulcers.
- It may also be used to stimulate movement of the stomach and intestines in cases of intestinal stoppage.

Are There Conditions or Times When Its Use Might Cause More Harm Than Good?

- Ranitidine should be used carefully in animals with heart disease as it may cause irregular heart beats in these animals if given by injection.
- Ranitidine should also be used carefully in animals with liver and kidney disease as the drug is removed from the body by these organs and may accumulate if these organs are not working properly.
- Ranitidine may cause increases in liver enzymes indicating damage to the liver. If your pet is going to receive ranitidine for a long time at a high dose, your veterinarian will want you to come back into the clinic frequently to have its liver checked.
- If your animal has any of the above conditions, talk to your veterinarian about the potential risks of using the medication versus the benefits that it might have.

What Side Effects Can Be Seen With Its Use?

- There are few side effects associated with ranitidine but some animals may experience diarrhea due to the stimulant effect on the intestines. Some animals may also have an irregular heartbeat and pain at the injection site when ranitidine is injected. If your pet experiences these side effects, contact your veterinarian.

How Should It Be Given?

- Ranitidine should be given on an empty stomach as giving with food will cause acid secretion before the drug starts to work.
- The successful outcome of your animal's treatment with this medication depends upon your commitment and ability to administer it exactly as the veterinarian has prescribed. Please do not skip doses or stop giving the medication. If you have difficulty giving doses consult your veterinarian or pharmacist who can offer administration techniques or change the dosage form to a type of medication that may be more acceptable to you and your animal.
- If you miss a dose of this medication you should give it as soon as you remember it, but if it is within a few hours of the regularly scheduled dose, wait and give it at the regular time. Do not double a dose as this can be toxic to your pet.
- Some other drugs can interact with this medication so tell your veterinarian about any drugs or foods that you currently give your animal. Do not give new foods or medications without first asking your veterinarian.
- **Dogs and Cats:** Dogs and cats usually receive this drug orally two to three times daily.
- **Horses:** Horses usually receive this medication orally three times daily. If the human tablets are used, it will take several tablets (10-12 of the 300mg tablets) per dose. Your pharmacist may be able to compound a paste or flavored suspension to get your horse to accept the medication more easily. It can be given with feed. Ranitidine is considered a Class 5 Drug by the Association of Racing Commissioners International (ARCI).

What Other Information Is Important About This Medication?

- Ranitidine tablets and liquid should be stored in a tight, light resistant, childproof container away from all children and other household pets.

Rifampin

Rifadin® and Rimactane® are other names for this medication.

How Is This Medication Useful?

- Rifampin is an antibiotic used to treat certain kinds of infections in animals. It is usually used for infections involving the lungs.

Are There Conditions or Times When Its Use Might Cause More Harm Than Good?

- Rifampin should not be used in animals that are allergic to it or to drugs like it. You should give rifampin regularly and not skip any doses as irregular dosing may increase the risk of an allergic reaction to rifampin.
- Rifampin is removed from the body by the liver and should be used at lower doses, if at all, in animals with liver disease.
- Rifampin should not be used alone as an antibiotic. It is easier for the bacteria become resistant to it when used alone.
- Rifampin has caused birth defects at high doses in laboratory animals, but it has been used safely in pregnant humans.
- You should always give all of the medication as directed by your veterinarian. If the entire course of treatment is not finished, the germ causing the infection may become stronger than the antibiotics and cause a worsening infection.
- If your animal has any of the above conditions, talk to your veterinarian about the potential risks of using the medication versus the benefits that it might have.

What Side Effects Can Be Seen With Its Use?

- Rifampin most commonly will cause the body secretions (tears, saliva, urine) to become orange. This is normal and harmless to the animal although it may cause permanent stains on carpet and furniture. Touching the drug will also stain human skin and will not easily wash off.
- Some animals given the drug have developed rashes.
- Many animals will develop stomach upset with rifampin. It should still be given on an empty stomach to make sure that it gets into the bloodstream.
- Rifampin may cause an increase in liver enzymes and your veterinarian will want to watch your pet's liver while taking this medication.
- The action of rifampin affects or is affected by many other drugs. You should tell your veterinarian about any other drugs that you are giving your pet.

How Should It Be Given?

- Rifampin should be given orally once or twice daily as directed by your veterinarian. It should be given on an empty stomach for complete effect. If you open the capsules or handle the oral liquid, it will likely stain your skin orange. This stain is harmless (unless you are allergic to rifampin) but will be difficult to wash off. You should wear gloves when handling this medication to avoid staining. Oral liquids of rifampin will need to be shaken well and kept in the refrigerator.
- Your veterinarian will prescribe another antibiotic (usually erythromycin) to use with the rifampin. Do not give one without the other as it may cause the bacteria to become resistant to the rifampin.
- The successful outcome of your animal's treatment with this medication depends upon your commitment and ability to administer it exactly as the veterinarian has prescribed. Please do not skip doses or stop giving the medication. If you have difficulty giving doses consult your veterinarian or pharmacist who can offer administration techniques or change the dosage form to a type of medication that may be more acceptable to you and your animal.
- If you miss a dose of this medication you should give it as soon as you remember it, but if it is within a few hours of the regularly scheduled dose, wait and give it at the regular time. Do not double a dose as this can be toxic to your pet.
- Some other drugs can interact with this medication so tell your veterinarian about any drugs or foods that you currently give your animal. Do not give new foods or medications without first asking your veterinarian.
- **Dogs and Cats**: Rifampin is usually given orally as a liquid or a capsule once to three times daily.
- **Horses**: Adult horses rarely receive rifampin, but foals receive it orally three times daily usually along with another antibiotic (erythromycin). You should increase the dose as directed by your veterinarian as your foal gains weight to make sure it is getting an adequate dose.

What Other Information Is Important About This Medication?

- Rifampin should be stored in a tight, light resistant, childproof container away from all children and other household pets. Oral liquids should be shaken well and stored in the refrigerator.
- Disposable gloves should be worn when handling or giving this drug to animals as this medication can stain skin and can cause rashes in people.
- You should make sure your pet has plenty of opportunity to use the litter box or eliminate outside as rifampin turns urine orange and this orange urine will stain carpets and furniture.

Selegilene

Anipryl®, Eldepryl® and l-deprenyl are other names for this medication.

How Is This Medication Useful?

- Selegilene is mostly used to treat confusion (dementia) caused by old age in animals. It is also used to treat some kinds of Cushing's Disease in dogs.

Are There Conditions or Times When Its Use Might Cause More Harm Than Good?

- Selegilene should not be used in animals that are allergic or are allergic to drugs like it.
- Selegilene inhibits an enzyme in the body called monoamine oxidase (MAO). When combined with certain drugs, it can cause serious (even fatal) increases in blood pressure. Aged cheese can also cause this effect, so make sure that your pets do not get into any aged cheese while on this drug. It should not be given with 5 weeks after drugs such as fluoxetine (Prozac®), phenylpropanolamine, some narcotic pain killers (Demerol®), or amitriptyline (Elavil®). Also, selegilene should be stopped for at least 2 weeks before any of these other drugs are started. You should tell your veterinarian about any medication or unusual food that you give your pet.
- Although laboratory studies have not shown any birth defects, selegilene should probably not be used in pregnant animals until further information is available.
- If your animal has any of the above conditions, talk to your veterinarian about the potential risks of using the medication versus the benefits that it might have.

What Side Effects Can Be Seen With Its Use?

- Some animals may experience loss of appetite, excessive drooling, stomach upset (vomiting or diarrhea), tiredness, confusion, loss of hearing and trembling.
- Some animals may develop itching.
- Other animals may develop repetitive behaviors such as walking in circles or becoming obsessed with something they ordinarily would not be interested in.
- If your animal's eyes are slow to respond to changes in light (pupils do not get smaller in bright light) or your animal is panting excessively, it may be overdosed and you should take your pet to a veterinarian immediately as this can be life-threatening.

How Should It Be Given?

- The successful outcome of your animal's treatment with this medication depends upon your commitment and ability to administer it exactly as the veterinarian has prescribed. Please do not skip doses or stop giving the medication. If you have difficulty giving doses consult your veterinarian or pharmacist who can offer administration techniques or change the dosage form to a type of medication that may be more acceptable to you and your animal.
- If you miss a dose of this medication you should give it as soon as you remember it, but if it is within a few hours of the regularly scheduled dose, wait and give it at the regular time. Do not double a dose as this can be toxic to your pet.
- Some other drugs can interact with this medication so tell your veterinarian about any drugs or foods that you currently give your animal. Do not give new foods or medications without first asking your veterinarian.
- **Dogs and Cats**: Selegilene should be given orally once daily in the morning for dogs and in the evening if used in cats. You should not give aged cheese or use tick collars while your pet is taking this medication.
- **Horses**: Selegilene probably does not work for the type of Cushing's disease that horses get.

What Other Information Is Important About This Medication?

- Selegilene should be stored in a tight, light resistant, childproof container away from all children and other household pets.

Sotalol

Betapace® is another name for this medication.

How Is This Medication Useful?

- Sotalol is a drug used to regulate your pet's heartbeat when a condition known as ventricular tachycardia exists.

Are There Conditions or Times When Its Use Might Cause More Harm Than Good?

- Sotalol should be used carefully, if at all, in animals with heart failure.
- Sotalol should not be used if your animal has a very slow heartbeat, asthma or other lung diseases.
- Sotalol is removed from the body by the kidneys and should be used carefully in patients with kidney disease.
- Sotalol can mask the signs of low blood sugar. It should be used very carefully in pets with diabetes. If your diabetic pet receives sotalol, your veterinarian should tell you exactly what to watch for to make sure that it is not getting dangerously low blood sugar levels.
- Sotalol may also mask the signs of an overactive thyroid and should be used carefully, if at all, in patients with hyperthyroidism (overactive thyroid).
- Several drugs will affect or be affected by sotalol. You should tell your veterinarian about any medications that you are giving your pet.
- If your animal has any of the above conditions, talk to your veterinarian about the potential risks of using the medication versus the benefits that it might have.

What Side Effects Can Be Seen With Its Use?

- Sotalol usually does not have many side effects when used properly.
- Some animals may develop a very slow heartbeat, become more tired and have lower blood pressure than usual.
- Rarely, animals may have difficulty breathing or vomit when taking this medication.

How Should It Be Given?

- Sotalol should preferably be given on an empty stomach (one hour before or two hours after feeding) as food can interfere with the drug's absorption.
- The successful outcome of your animal's treatment with this medication depends upon your commitment and ability to administer it exactly as the veterinarian has prescribed. Please do not skip doses or stop giving the medication. If you have difficulty giving doses consult your veterinarian or pharmacist who can offer administration techniques or change the dosage form to a type of medication that may be more acceptable to you and your animal.
- If you miss a dose of this medication you should give it as soon as you remember it, but if it is within a few hours of the regularly scheduled dose, wait and give it at the regular time. Do not double a dose as this can be toxic to your pet.
- Some other drugs can interact with this medication so tell your veterinarian about any drugs or foods that you currently give your animal. Do not give new foods or medications without first asking your veterinarian.
- **Dogs and Cats**: Dogs usually receive sotalol orally one to two times daily. Cats usually don't receive sotalol
- **Horses**: Horses don't usually receive sotalol.

What Other Information Is Important About This Medication?

- Sotalol should be stored at room temperature in a tight, light resistant, childproof container away from all children and other household pets.
- Sotalol treatment can be quite expensive.

VETERINARY DRUG HANDBOOK-Client Information Edition
Permission to photocopy for individual clients granted by Gigi Davidson and Donald C. Plumb © 2003

Spironolactone

Aldactone® is another name for this medication.

How Is This Medication Useful?

- Spironolactone is a diuretic that is used in patients who don't respond to other diuretics or who have developed a low potassium from other diuretics. Spironlactone does not cause loss of potassium like other diuretics (furosemide-Lasix®).

Are There Conditions or Times When Its Use Might Cause More Harm Than Good?

- Spironolactone causes the body to save potassium. It should not be used in animals that already have too much potassium or where increased potassium levels could cause problems (Addison's Disease, diabetes).
- Spironolactone should be used with extreme caution in animals with liver or kidney disease.
- Spironolactone inactivates the drug called mitotane which is used to treat Cushing's Disease in dogs. You should not give spironolactone to a dog who is being treated with mitotane.
- If your animal has any of the above conditions, talk to your veterinarian about the potential risks of using the medication versus the benefits that it might have.

What Side Effects Can Be Seen With Its Use?

- Spironolactone can cause high levels of potassium in the blood. If your animal becomes weak or lethargic (lacking energy) while on spironolactone, you should call your veterinarian.
- Spironolactone can cause loss of sodium from the blood and make your animal weak or confused. If you notice these signs, call your veterinarian.
- As spironolactone is a diuretic, it can cause too much water loss and your pet can become dehydrated. Make sure your pet has access to plenty of fresh, clean drinking water at all times.
- Some animals will get stomach upset (vomiting and diarrhea) from spironolactone.
- Some human males have developed breast enlargement from spironolactone. It is not known if this happens in male animals.
- Spironolactone is affected by or alters the effects of many other drugs. You should tell your veterinarian about all drugs that you give your pet.

How Should It Be Given?

- Spironolactone should be given orally once to twice daily. If the commercially available tablets are not appropriate for your pet, your veterinarian may instruct a pharmacist to compound a special oral liquid which is good for 30 days if stored in the refrigerator.
- The successful outcome of your animal's treatment with this medication depends upon your commitment and ability to administer it exactly as the veterinarian has prescribed. Please do not skip doses or stop giving the medication. If you have difficulty giving doses consult your veterinarian or pharmacist who can offer administration techniques or change the dosage form to a type of medication that may be more acceptable to you and your animal.
- If you miss a dose of this medication you should give it as soon as you remember it, but if it is within a few hours of the regularly scheduled dose, wait and give it at the regular time. Do not double a dose as this can be toxic to your pet.
- Some other drugs can interact with this medication so tell your veterinarian about any drugs or foods that you currently give your animal. Do not give new foods or medications without first asking your veterinarian.
- **Dogs and Cats**: Dogs and cats usually receive spironolactone orally once or twice daily.
- **Horses**: Spironolactone is not usually used in horses, but is considered a Class 4 Drug by the Association of Racing Commissioners International (ARCI).

What Other Information Is Important About This Medication?

- Spironolactone should be stored in a tight, light resistant, childproof container away from all children and other household pets.
- Specially compounded oral liquids of spironolactone should be shaken well, stored in the refrigerator, and discarded after 30 days.

Stanozolol

Winstrol® is another name for this medication.

How Is This Medication Useful?

- Stanozolol is an anabolic steroid that is used to improve appetite, cause weight gain, and increase muscle strength.
- It is also used to cause increased blood cell formation in anemia.

Are There Conditions or Times When Its Use Might Cause More Harm Than Good?

- Stanozolol should not be used in pregnant animals due to extreme adverse effects on the unborn babies.
- Stanozolol should not be used in male animals intending for breeding as it severely reduces sperm count.
- Stanozolol should not be used in animals that have cancer of the mammary glands (breasts) or prostate.
- Stanozolol can cause a severe liver disease in cats and should be used extremely carefully in this species.
- Stanozolol causes water retention and should not be used in patients with heart disease, kidney disease or patients being treated for diabetes insipidus.
- Stanozolol can also increase the amount of calcium in blood and may cause severe problems in patients who already have weak hearts.
- If your animal has any of the above conditions, talk to your veterinarian about the potential risks of using the medication versus the benefits that it might have.

What Side Effects Can Be Seen With Its Use?

- Stanozolol acts like a male hormone and can cause female animals to not come into heat. It may also make female animals exhibit male breeding behavior (mounting other animals.) It can also cause other behavior changes. If your pet shows any unusual behavior, contact your veterinarian for advice.
- Stanozolol can cause water retention and swelling.
- Stanozolol can cause increased calcium in the blood. If you notice that your pet seems unusually tired, weak, or has an irregular heartbeat, you should contact your veterinarian immediately.

How Should It Be Given?

- Stanozolol should be given with food orally once or twice daily. It may take several weeks to have the effect that your veterinarian wants.
- Stanozolol is a controlled substance and should only be given to the pet for whom the prescription was written.
- The successful outcome of your animal's treatment with this medication depends upon your commitment and ability to administer it exactly as the veterinarian has prescribed. Please do not skip doses or stop giving the medication. If you have difficulty giving doses consult your veterinarian or pharmacist who can offer administration techniques or change the dosage form to a type of medication that may be more acceptable to you and your animal.
- If you miss a dose of this medication you should give it as soon as you remember it, but if it is within a few hours of the regularly scheduled dose, wait and give it at the regular time. Do not double a dose as this can be toxic to your pet.
- Some other drugs can interact with this medication so tell your veterinarian about any drugs or foods that you currently give your animal. Do not give new foods or medications without first asking your veterinarian.
- **Dogs and Cats**: Stanozolol is given orally to dogs once or twice daily. It may also be given by injection once weekly. It is rarely used in cats but when used is given orally once daily.
- **Horses**: Horses usually receive stanozolol by injection once weekly. It is considered a Class 4 drug by the Association of Racing Commissioners International (ARCI).

What Other Information Is Important About This Medication?

- Stanozolol should be stored in a tight, light resistant, childproof container away from all children and other household pets. The injection should be shaken thoroughly before using.
- Stanozolol is a controlled substance. You will need to get a new prescription for this medication every 6 months and you should not give it to any other pets.

Sucralfate

Carafate® is another name for this medication.

How Is This Medication Useful?

- Sucralfate is used to coat ulcers in the stomach to protect them from further damage. It is also used to prevent the formation of ulcers. It will coat the ulcer for up to 6 hours after an oral dose.

Are There Conditions or Times When Its Use Might Cause More Harm Than Good?

- Sucralfate might worsen constipation and should not be used in conditions where slowing the action of the stomach and intestines could be harmful (e.g., megacolon).
- Sucralfate contains aluminum. Long term use may cause higher levels of aluminum to accumulate and weaken the bones or have an effect on the brain.
- Sucralfate has caused no deformities in pregnant laboratory animals, but until further information is available, it should be used cautiously in pregnant animals.
- Sucralfate binds many drugs in the stomach and prevents them from having an effect. Tell your veterinarian if you are giving your pets any other medications and don't give any medications within 2 hours of sucralfate.
- If your animal has any of the above conditions, talk to your veterinarian about the potential risks of using the medication versus the benefits that it might have.

What Side Effects Can Be Seen With Its Use?

- Constipation is generally the only side effect seen with sucralfate.

How Should It Be Given?

- Sucralfate should be given orally up to 4 times daily. If giving the tablets, they should ideally be crushed before administration to give maximum ulcer protection. Liquid forms of sucralfate cover ulcers better than whole tablets.
- The successful outcome of your animal's treatment with this medication depends upon your commitment and ability to administer it exactly as the veterinarian has prescribed. Please do not skip doses or stop giving the medication. If you have difficulty giving doses consult your veterinarian or pharmacist who can offer administration techniques or change the dosage form to a type of medication that may be more acceptable to you and your animal.

- If you miss a dose of this medication you should give it as soon as you remember it, but if it is within a few hours of the regularly scheduled dose, wait and give it at the regular time. Do not double a dose as this can be toxic to your pet.
- Some other drugs can interact with this medication so tell your veterinarian about any drugs or foods that you currently give your animal. Do not give new foods or medications without first asking your veterinarian.
- **Dogs and Cats**: Dogs and cats usually receive sucralfate as an oral liquid or as crushed tablets 2-4 times daily on an empty stomach. Oral liquids should be shaken well before giving. Other drugs should not be given within 2 hours of sucralfate.
- **Horses**: Horses receive sucralfate orally four times daily. Crushing the tablets increases their protective effect. Sucralfate tablets dissolve very rapidly and easily in lukewarm water which may make it easier to give sucralfate orally to your horse.

What Other Information Is Important About This Medication?

- Sucralfate should be stored in a tight, light resistant, childproof container away from all children and other household pets.
- You should watch your animal for continued signs that sucralfate is working. If you see blood in the vomit or stools, or your horse is grinding its teeth, you should contact your veterinarian immediately as the ulcers may be getting worse.

Sulfasalazine

Azulfidine® is another name for this medication.

How Is This Medication Useful?

- Sulfasalazine is a sulfa drug that is used to treat bowel disorders where inflammation is the cause.

Are There Conditions or Times When Its Use Might Cause More Harm Than Good?

- Sulfasalazine is a sulfa and may cause allergic reactions in pets and owners who are allergic to sulfa drugs.
- Sulfasalazine contains an aspirin-like substance. It may cause allergies in pets and owners who are allergic to aspirin. Since aspirin can be very toxic to cats, this drug should be monitored very carefully when used in cats.
- Sulfas should not be used in animals that are dehydrated as stone formation may occur in the kidneys. Always make sure that your pet has plenty of fresh, clean drinking water while on sulfa drugs
- Sulfa drugs can cause a decrease in tear production in dogs (dry-eye) and should probably not be used in dogs that already have dry-eye. It should also be used with caution in breeds that are pre-disposed to dry-eye.
- This drug has not been shown to cause birth defects but should be used carefully in pregnancy and probably not at all in the first trimester of pregnancy.
- Sulfa drugs can cause anemia and should not be used in animals that currently have or have had anemia.
- Sulfasalazine may reduce sperm count and should be used with caution in males that are intended for breeding.
- Sulfasalazine is removed from the body by the liver and the kidneys and should not be used in animals that have liver or kidney disease.
- If your animal has any of the above conditions, talk to your veterinarian about the potential risks of using the medication versus the benefits that it might have.

What Side Effects Can Be Seen With Its Use?

- Some dogs will develop dry-eye from sulfa drugs. If you notice your dog squinting, blinking more, rubbing its eyes, or notice that it has more eye discharge than usual, you should contact your veterinarian immediately.
- Many cats will develop loss of appetite and vomiting from sulfasalazine.

- Trimethoprim and sulfa drugs can suppress the bone marrow and cause anemia. If you notice fever (103-105°F) or unusual tiredness in your dog or cat, you should contact your veterinarian. These drugs should probably not be used if your animal has a history of severe anemia.
- Sulfa drugs may rarely cause a severe skin condition that can cause significant loss of skin. If you notice unusual itching or any skin inflammation while your pet is taking sulfa drugs, you should contact your veterinarian immediately.
- Sulfas should not be used in animals that are dehydrated as stone formation may occur in the kidneys. Always make sure that your pet has plenty of fresh, clean drinking water while on sulfa drugs.

How Should It Be Given?

- Sulfasalazine should be given with food orally up to three times daily. Your veterinarian may gradually increase the dose until the diarrhea resolves. Once stools are normal, the dose may gradually be decreased to the lowest effective dose.
- The successful outcome of your animal's treatment with this medication depends upon your commitment and ability to administer it exactly as the veterinarian has prescribed. Please do not skip doses or stop giving the medication. If you have difficulty giving doses consult your veterinarian or pharmacist who can offer administration techniques or change the dosage form to a type of medication that may be more acceptable to you and your animal.
- If you miss a dose of this medication you should give it as soon as you remember it, but if it is within a few hours of the regularly scheduled dose, wait and give it at the regular time. Do not double a dose as this can be toxic to your pet.
- Some other drugs can interact with this medication so tell your veterinarian about any drugs or foods that you currently give your animal. Do not give new foods or medications without first asking your veterinarian.
- **Dogs and Cats**: Dogs usually receive sulfasalazine two to three times daily while cats receive it once daily. Dosage may be adjusted downward to the lowest effective dose once the diarrhea goes away.

What Other Information Is Important About This Medication?

- Sulfasalazine should be stored in a tight, light resistant, childproof container away from all children and other household pets.

Taurine

2-aminosulphonic acid is another name for this medication.

How Is This Medication Useful?

- Taurine is an essential amino acid that protects the retina of the eye as well as the heart muscle in dogs and cats. Cats cannot make taurine from other proteins so they must receive it in their diet. It is present in most commercially available pet foods but some animals will still develop a deficiency. It is given as a supplement to help animals with eye and heart disease. It may also be used to reduce seizures in cats and dogs.

Are There Conditions or Times When Its Use Might Cause More Harm Than Good?

- Although taurine does not require a prescription, it should not be used unless your veterinarian has prescribed it for your pet.

What Side Effects Can Be Seen With Its Use?

- There have been some cases of stomach upset with taurine, but side effects are rare.

How Should It Be Given?

- Taurine may be given orally or mixed in the food once to twice daily.
- The successful outcome of your animal's treatment with this medication depends upon your commitment and ability to administer it exactly as the veterinarian has prescribed. Please do not skip doses or stop giving the medication. If you have difficulty giving doses consult your veterinarian or pharmacist who can offer administration techniques or change the dosage form to a type of medication that may be more acceptable to you and your animal.

- If you miss a dose of this medication you should give it as soon as you remember it, but if it is within a few hours of the regularly scheduled dose, wait and give it at the regular time. Do not double a dose as this can be toxic to your pet.
- Some other drugs can interact with this medication so tell your veterinarian about any drugs or foods that you currently give your animal. Do not give new foods or medications without first asking your veterinarian.
- **Dogs and Cats**: Dogs and cats usually receive taurine orally once or twice daily.
- **Horses**: Horses do not usually receive taurine.

What Other Information Is Important About This Medication?

- Taurine should be stored in a tight, light resistant, childproof container away from all children and other household pets.
- It may be purchased without a prescription at health and nutrition stores as a tablet or a capsule ranging in size from 125-500mg.

Terbutaline

Brethine® and Bricanyl® are other names for this medication.

How Is This Medication Useful?

- Terbutaline is a drug that dilates the lung passages to allow air to get into the lungs of animals with asthma or other respiratory diseases.
- It is also sometimes injected under the skin to diagnose a condition called anhydrosis in horses; a condition where they cannot sweat.

Are There Conditions or Times When Its Use Might Cause More Harm Than Good?

- Terbutaline should not be used in animals who are known to be allergic to it and drugs like it.
- Terbutaline speeds up the heart and should not be used in animals with heart disease.
- Terbutaline should be used with caution, if at all, in patients with overactive thyroid, diabetes, seizures, and high blood pressure.
- Terbutaline should not be used in pregnant animals.
- If your animal has any of the above conditions, talk to your veterinarian about the potential risks of using the medication versus the benefits that it might have.

What Side Effects Can Be Seen With Its Use?

- Terbutaline can speed up the heart and cause a racing heart beat. If your animal's pulse is consistently over 200 while taking terbutaline, you should contact your veterinarian.
- Terbutaline also causes trembling, shakiness, nervousness, vomiting and diarrhea.
- Terbutaline may decrease the amount of potassium in the blood. Call your veterinarian if your animal shows signs of weakness or muscle trembling.
- Terbutaline affects or is affected by many other drugs. Tell your veterinarian about any drugs that your pet may be receiving before giving terbutaline.

How Should It Be Given?

- The successful outcome of your animal's treatment with this medication depends upon your commitment and ability to administer it exactly as the veterinarian has prescribed. Please do not skip doses or stop giving the medication. If you have difficulty giving doses consult your veterinarian or pharmacist who can offer administration techniques or change the dosage form to a type of medication that may be more acceptable to you and your animal.
- If you miss a dose of this medication you should give it as soon as you remember it, but if it is within a few hours of the regularly scheduled dose, wait and give it at the regular time. Do not double a dose as this can be toxic to your pet.
- Some other drugs can interact with this medication so tell your veterinarian about any drugs or foods that you currently give your animal. Do not give new foods or medications without first asking your veterinarian.
- **Dogs and Cats**: Dogs and cats usually receive this medication orally two to three times daily.
- **Horses**: It may be injected under your horse's skin in varying amounts to see if your horse can sweat properly. It is considered a Class 3 drug by the Association of Racing Commissioners International (ARCI).

What Other Information Is Important About This Medication?

- Terbutaline should be stored in a tight, light resistant, childproof container away from all children and other household pets.

Tetracycline

Panmycin® and Sumycin® are other names for this medication.

How Is This Medication Useful?

- Tetracycline is used to treat many infections in pet, especially those diseases caused by ticks.

Are There Conditions or Times When Its Use Might Cause More Harm Than Good?

- Some animals are allergic to tetracycline. If your animal has shown allergies to any of the tetracycline products, you should tell your veterinarian before you give your pet tetracycline.
- Because animals do not swallow their medications with water, and because their bodies are horizontal instead of vertical, tablets and capsules can sometimes get stuck on their way to the stomach. You should ensure that your pet swallows some water after giving tetracycline.
- You should always give all of the medication as directed by your veterinarian. If the entire course of treatment is not finished, the germ causing the infection may become stronger than the antibiotics and cause a worsening infection.
- If your animal has any of the above conditions, talk to your veterinarian about the potential risks of using the medication versus the benefits that it might have.

What Side Effects Can Be Seen With Its Use?

- Nausea and vomiting are the most common side effects seen with dogs and cats given tetracycline. To reduce these side effects, give each dose with a meal. If your dog or cat experiences severe vomiting or diarrhea, contact your veterinarian.
- Tetracycline can also increase the sensitivity of the skin to sunlight. If your pet is light skinned, light furred or has thin fur, you should not let it go out into direct sunlight for more than a few minutes while taking tetracycline. Some sunscreens may be toxic to pets, so you should ask your veterinarian before putting any sunscreen on your animal.

How Should It Be Given?

- Tetracycline should be given on an empty stomach. It is inactivated by iron, milk products and antacids. You should make sure your pet drinks some water (never milk) to wash the medication down into its stomach. The successful outcome of your animal's treatment with this medication depends upon your commitment and ability to administer it exactly as the veterinarian has prescribed. Please do not skip doses or stop giving the medication. If you have difficulty giving doses consult your veterinarian or pharmacist who can offer administration techniques or change the dosage form to a type of medication that may be more acceptable to you and your animal.
- Some other drugs can interact with this medication so tell your veterinarian about any drugs or foods that you currently give your animal. Do not give new foods or medications without first asking your veterinarian.
- **Dogs and Cats**: Dogs and cats usually receive tetracycline orally twice or three times daily. Cats should be given at least a teaspoonful of water or offered a favorite liquid (not milk) to drink following tablets or capsules.
- **Horses**: Horses typically do not receive tetracycline orally as it can cause some problems with the gastrointestinal tract, however it is occasionally used to treat tick-borne diseases in horses.

What Other Information Is Important About This Medication?

- Pets should be watched carefully if they spend a lot of time in direct sunlight as tetracycline can cause the skin to erupt in pustules and blisters when exposed to sunlight.
- You should never give your pet "old" (expired) tetracycline as it breaks down to a product that can severely damage the kidneys.

Theophylline

Slo-bid®, Theobid®, Slo-Phyllin®, Theolair® are among the other names for this medication. Aminophylline and theophylline are equivalent drugs except dosages are figured differently.

How Is This Medication Useful?

• This medication is used to relax airways and help animals breathe better. It is used in conditions such as asthma or heaves. It is sometimes used with other medications in the treatment of symptoms of heart failure.

Are There Conditions or Times When Its Use Might Cause More Harm Than Good?

• Theophylline can cause the heart to beat too fast. It should be used with extreme caution in animals with irregular heartbeats or heart disease.

• Theophylline might also worsen the conditions of stomach ulcers, thyroid disease, kidney or liver disease or high blood pressure.

• Theophylline might take longer to get out of the bodies of very young or very old animals and should be used carefully in these patients.

• If your animal has any of the above conditions, talk to your veterinarian about the potential risks of using the medication versus the benefits that it might have.

What Side Effects Can Be Seen With Its Use?

• The most common side effects from theophylline are stomach upset and fast heartbeat. At the beginning of treatment, your animal may experience nervousness and stomach upset but these side effects usually go away as your animal's body gets used to the medication.

• Theophylline may cause some animals to eat more, drink more and urinate more.

• Horses may become more nervous, have a fast heartbeat, sweat and be unstable on their feet.

• In higher doses, some animals may have seizures.

• If you see any of these side effects in your animal, you should tell your veterinarian immediately.

How Should It Be Given?

• Theophylline should be given exactly as your veterinarian has told you. It can be dangerous in doses that are too high. You should never skip doses. If you accidentally forget to give a dose, you should never double the next dose to make up for it.

• The successful outcome of your animal's treatment with this medication depends upon your commitment and ability to administer it exactly as the veterinarian has prescribed. If you have difficulty giving any doses, please do not skip doses or stop giving the medication.

• Consult your veterinarian or pharmacist who can offer administration techniques or change the dosage form to a type of medication that may be more acceptable to you and your animal.

• Some other drugs can interact with this medication so tell your veterinarian about any drugs or foods that you currently give your animal. Do not give new foods or medications without first asking your veterinarian.

• **Dogs and Cats**: Theophylline is usually given to dogs and cats twice or three times daily. It should be given exactly as the veterinarian has instructed. You should not crush tablets of long-acting theophylline as this may release too much drug into your pet's bloodstream at once and cause severe adverse effects. It is not unusual at the beginning of treatment for animals to experience nervousness or upset stomach from this drug. These side effects should go away in a short time. If these effects return after a while, you should tell your veterinarian immediately.

• **Horses**: This drug is banned for use in horses that are going to show or race. It is usually given two or three times daily and may be mixed in the feed. Horses may initially show nervousness, sweating, and fast heartbeat and may be unstable on their feet. These side effects will usually go away with time.

What Other Information Is Important About This Medication?

• This medication should be stored at room temperature and protected from extreme heat or freezing.

• **Horses**: This drug is banned by the ASHA and should not be used in show or race horses while they are performing.

• There are many different brands of long-acting theophylline. You should contact your veterinarian before switching brands once your animal is controlled. If you do receive a brand that your pet has not taken before, you should watch it for signs of adverse effects and take your pet to the clinic if necessary.

Trimeprazine with Prednisolone

Temaril-P® is another name for this medication.

How Is This Medication Useful?

- Trimeprazine and prednisolone is an antihistamine-glucocorticoid combination used to treat severe itching in animals. It may also be useful as a cough suppressant.

Are There Conditions or Times When Its Use Might Cause More Harm Than Good?

- Because Temaril-P® has a glucorticoid (steroid) in it, it should not be used in respiratory infections without an antibiotic to control the infection. Steroids can often worsen infections as they suppress the immune system.
- Steroids (e.g., prednisolone) should never be used in the presence of fungal infection as these drugs will make the fungal infection much worse.
- Animals with Cushing's disease already make too much glucocorticoid (steroid) and this drug should not be used in those animals.
- Steroids should not be used in diabetic animals or pregnant animals.
- Trimeprazine is an antihistamine of the type that has been known to cause seizures in animals prone to having them. If your pet has ever had a seizure, you should let your veterinarian know before using this drug.
- If your animal has any of the above conditions, talk to your veterinarian about the potential risks of using the medication versus the benefits that it might have.

What Side Effects Can Be Seen With Its Use?

- Drowsiness is a common side effect from antihistamines.
- Trimeprazine may also cause muscle tremors, rigidity and restlessness.
- Animals treated with prednisolone will have increased appetite, increased thirst and an increased need to urinate. You should be aware that your pet may need to go out more frequently to urinate. As it is stressful to some pets to have "accidents" you should make sure that your pet can go outside or have a clean litter box when needed.
- Glucocorticoid drugs will suppress your animal's immune system and may increase the risk for infection. If your pet shows any signs of fever (103-105°F in most dogs and cats), or acts like it

has a urinary tract infection (frequent or painful urination) you should contact your veterinarian immediately.

- Some animals on long-term therapy with prednisolone will develop Cushing's disease. If your pet shows signs of dry hair coat or hair loss, weakness and muscle loss, darkening of the skin, or develops a pot-belly, you should contact your veterinarian.
- Some animals may become aggressive while on prednisolone. You should contact your veterinarian if this behavior change occurs or does not go away with time.
- Prednisolone will cause changes in your pet's insulin requirements if it is a diabetic. You should ask your veterinarian for instructions on how to deal with these changes if your pet is receiving insulin injections.

How Should It Be Given?

- Trimeprazine and prednisolone should be given orally with food to reduce the chances of stomach ulcers or irritation. If given once daily, trimeprazine and prednisolone is usually given in the morning to dogs, and in the evening to cats as this will more closely mimic their natural hormone cycles.
- The successful outcome of your animal's treatment with this medication depends upon your commitment and ability to administer it exactly as the veterinarian has prescribed. Please do not skip doses or stop giving the medication. If you have difficulty giving doses consult your veterinarian or pharmacist who can offer administration techniques or change the dosage form to a type of medication that may be more acceptable to you and your animal.
- If you miss a dose of this medication you should give it as soon as you remember it, but if it is within a few hours of the regularly scheduled dose, wait and give it at the regular time. Do not double a dose as this can be toxic to your pet.
- Some other drugs can interact with this medication so tell your veterinarian about any drugs or foods that you currently give your animal. Do not give new foods or medications without first asking your veterinarian.
- **Dogs**: Dogs usually receive this drug orally twice daily with food.

What Other Information Is Important About This Medication?

- Trimeprazine and prednisolone should be stored in a tight, light resistant, childproof container away from all children and other household pets.

Trimethoprim with Sulfamethoxazole or Sulfadiazine

Tribrissen®, Tucoprim®, Septra® and Bactrim® are other names for this medication.

How Is This Medication Useful?
- Trimethoprim sulfa combinations are strong antibiotics used to treat infections in animals.

Are There Conditions or Times When Its Use Might Cause More Harm Than Good?
- Trimethoprim/Sulfa combinations should not be used in animals who are known to be allergic to sulfa drugs. Humans with sulfa allergies should also avoid contact with this drug.
- These drugs should probably not be used if your animal has a history of severe anemia.
- Trimethoprim sulfa combinations should not be used in animals with severe liver or kidney diseases as the drug can worsen these conditions.
- Trimethoprim and sulfa drugs inhibit the brain development of growing fetuses. It should not be used in pregnant animals.
- Sulfa drugs should not be used in animals who have kidney stones or have had kidney stones as these drugs may worsen stone formation.
- Sulfas should not be used in animals that are dehydrated as stone formation may occur in the kidneys. Always make sure that your pet has plenty of fresh, clean drinking water while on sulfa drugs.
- You should always give all of the medication as directed by your veterinarian. If the entire course of treatment is not finished, the germ causing the infection may become stronger than the antibiotics and cause a worsening infection.
- If your animal has any of the above conditions, talk to your veterinarian about the potential risks of using the medication versus the benefits that it might have.

What Side Effects Can Be Seen With Its Use?
- Some dogs will develop dry eye (keratoconjunctivitis sicca) from sulfa drugs. If your dog starts blinking more, rubbing its eyes or has lots of eye discharge, you should contact your veterinarian immediately.
- Some animals will develop stomach upset (vomiting and diarrhea) from trimethoprim sulfa combinations.

- Some animals may develop an arthritis like condition while on sulfa drugs.
- Trimethoprim and sulfa drugs can suppress the bone marrow and cause anemia. If you notice fever (103-105°F) or unusual tiredness in your dog or cat, you should contact your veterinarian. These drugs should probably not be used if your animal has a history of severe anemia.
- Sulfas should not be used in animals that are dehydrated as stone formation may occur in the kidneys. Always make sure that your pet has plenty of fresh, clean drinking water while on sulfa drugs.
- Some horses will get a very bad (sometimes fatal) diarrhea from paste forms of this drug given orally.
- Sulfa drugs may rarely cause a severe skin condition that can cause significant loss of skin. If you notice unusual itching or any skin inflammation while your pet is taking sulfa drugs, you should contact your veterinarian immediately.
- Some dogs will develop an underactive thyroid on this medication if given longer than 6 weeks.

How Should It Be Given?
- This drug should be given with plenty of fresh water to help prevent the side effects that are worsened by dehydration.
- The successful outcome of your animal's treatment with this medication depends upon your commitment and ability to administer it exactly as the veterinarian has prescribed. Please do not skip doses or stop giving the medication. If you have difficulty giving doses consult your veterinarian or pharmacist who can offer administration techniques or change the dosage form to a type of medication that may be more acceptable to you and your animal.
- If you miss a dose of this medication you should give it as soon as you remember it, but if it is within a few hours of the regularly scheduled dose, wait and give it at the regular time. Do not double a dose as this can be toxic to your pet.

(Continued on following page)

(continued)

How Should It Be Given?
(continued from previous page)

- Some other drugs can interact with this medication so tell your veterinarian about any drugs or foods that you currently give your animal. Do not give new foods or medications without first asking your veterinarian.

- **Dogs and Cats**: Dogs and cats usually receive trimethoprim sulfa combinations orally once or twice daily. Cats are repulsed by the taste of trimethoprim sulfa combinations and will salivate profusely if allowed to taste it. Providing trimethoprim sulfa combinations to cats in capsules or other dosage forms that will prevent direct contact with the tongue will make administration of this drug much more pleasant for both the cat and the owner.

- **Horses**: Horses usually receive this medication orally once or twice daily. Oral paste formulations of this drug have caused severe diarrheas in some horses. If your horse develops diarrhea while on this medication you should contact your veterinarian immediately for advice.

What Other Information Is Important About This Medication?

- Trimethoprim sulfa combinations should be stored in a tight, light resistant, childproof container away from all children and other household pets.
- Oral liquids of trimethoprim sulfa should be shaken well before use.

Tylosin

Tylan® is another name for this medication.

How Is This Medication Useful?

- Tylosin is a macrolide antibiotic that is used to treat certain types of chronic diarrhea in dogs and cats.

Are There Conditions or Times When Its Use Might Cause More Harm Than Good?

- Tylosin should not be used in animals that are allergic to it or to other drugs like it.
- Tylosin should not be given to horses as it may kill all the helpful bacteria in their intestines and cause a fatal diarrhea.
- It is not known if tylosin can be used safely in pregnancy but there are no reports of adverse effects when used in pregnant animals.
- If your animal has any of the above conditions, talk to your veterinarian about the potential risks of using the medication versus the benefits that it might have.

What Side Effects Can Be Seen With Its Use?

- Some animals may have a mild stomach ache when first receiving tylosin and experience vomiting and an initial worsening of diarrhea.

How Should It Be Given?

- Tylosin should be given with food orally twice daily. The only products available are powdered formulations that are very bitter and may be rejected by the animal. Your veterinarian may instruct you how to administer the powder mixed in water or food or may have it compounded into oral capsules for an exact dose that may be more accepted by your animal. If you mix the powder with water, it must be made fresh every 3 days or it will break down and not be effective.
- The successful outcome of your animal's treatment with this medication depends upon your commitment and ability to administer it exactly as the veterinarian has prescribed. Please do not skip doses or stop giving the medication. If you have difficulty giving doses consult your veterinarian or pharmacist who can offer administration techniques or change the dosage form to a type of medication that may be more acceptable to you and your animal.
- If you miss a dose of this medication you should give it as soon as you remember it, but if it is within a few hours of the regularly scheduled dose, wait and give it at the regular time. Do not double a dose as this can be toxic to your pet.
- Some other drugs can interact with this medication so tell your veterinarian about any drugs or foods that you currently give your animal. Do not give new foods or medications without first asking your veterinarian.
- **Dogs and Cats**: Dogs and cats usually receive tylosin orally as a powder, liquid or capsule twice daily. If given as a liquid, solutions should be made fresh every 3 days.
- **Horses**: Tylosin should not be given orally to horses as it can cause a fatal diarrhea.

What Other Information Is Important About This Medication?

- Tylosin powder and capsules should be stored in a tight, light resistant, childproof container away from all children and other household pets.
- Tylosin liquids should be discarded every 3 days and fresh ones made.

VETERINARY DRUG HANDBOOK-Client Information Edition
Permission to photocopy for individual clients granted by Gigi Davidson and Donald C. Plumb © 2003

Ursodiol

Actigall® is another name for this medication.

How Is This Medication Useful?
- Ursodiol is a bile acid that is given orally to treat liver and gallbladder disease in cats.
- It may also be used to assist in removal of cholesterol containing gallstones.

Are There Conditions or Times When Its Use Might Cause More Harm Than Good?
- Ursodiol should not be used in rabbits and other animals that are hindgut fermenters as these species will turn ursodiol into a very toxic substance that will severely damage the liver.
- Animals receiving ursodiol should not receive acetaminophen (Tylenol®) or other drugs that are removed from the body by a process called sulfation. Tell your veterinarian about other drugs that your animal may be taking.
- Ursodiol should not be used in patients that have shown an allergy to it or other bile acid like drugs.
- Ursodiol may actually worsen liver function in some patients and should be discontinued if liver tests indicate that liver function is worsening.
- If your animal has any of the above conditions, talk to your veterinarian about the potential risks of using the medication versus the benefits that it might have.

What Side Effects Can Be Seen With Its Use?
- Ursodiol is generally well-tolerated in dogs and cats although some may experience diarrhea.
- Ursodiol will not dissolve existing gallstones and other measures must be undertaken to remove these stones.

How Should It Be Given?
- Ursodiol should be given orally once or twice daily with oil or a fatty meal.
- Because ursodiol is only available as a capsule for humans, your veterinarian may prescribe a compounded formulation to achieve the right dose for your animal. Ursodiol may be compounded into capsules which can be given with oil or sprinkled on food, or it may be compounded into an oral liquid in oil.

- The successful outcome of your animal's treatment with this medication depends upon your commitment and ability to administer it exactly as the veterinarian has prescribed. Please do not skip doses or stop giving the medication. If you have difficulty giving doses consult your veterinarian or pharmacist who can offer administration techniques or change the dosage form to a type of medication that may be more acceptable to you and your animal.
- If you miss a dose of this medication you should give it as soon as you remember it, but if it is within a few hours of the regularly scheduled dose, wait and give it at the regular time. Do not double a dose as this can be toxic to your pet.
- Some other drugs can interact with this medication so tell your veterinarian about any drugs or foods that you currently give your animal. Do not give new foods or medications without first asking your veterinarian.
- **Dogs and Cats**: Dogs and cats usually receive ursodiol orally with a fatty meal twice daily.
- **Horses**: Horses do not have gallbladders, so ursodiol would not be of any use in this species.
- **Rabbits/Guinea Pigs**: Ursodiol should not be used in these species as it is converted to a very toxic substance in their hindguts and will cause severe (fatal) liver damage.

What Other Information Is Important About This Medication?
- Ursodiol should be stored in a tight, light resistant, childproof container away from all children and other household pets.
- Liquid forms of ursodiol should be shaken well and discarded after about 35 days.
- Ursodiol should not be given with a drug called cholestyramine (Questran®) as it will completely bind up the drug and prevent it from working.

Vitamin E

Alpha tocopherol is another name for this medication.

How Is This Medication Useful?

- Vitamin E is an antioxidant used to protect cells and assists in fat metabolism. Deficiencies of Vitamin E will cause cell damage and death in skeletal muscle, heart, testes, liver, and nerves. It is also used to promote skin healing. It may also be used to support the treatment of horses with equine protozoal myeloencephalitis (EPM).

Are There Conditions or Times When Its Use Might Cause More Harm Than Good?

- Giving vitamin E by rapid injection may cause allergic reactions.
- If your animal has any of the above conditions, talk to your veterinarian about the potential risks of using the medication versus the benefits that it might have.

What Side Effects Can Be Seen With Its Use?

- There are no known side effects from vitamin E, even at extremely high doses.

How Should It Be Given?

- Vitamin E is a fat-soluble vitamin and should be given with a fatty meal to ensure complete absorption into the bloodstream.
- The successful outcome of your animal's treatment with this medication depends upon your commitment and ability to administer it exactly as the veterinarian has prescribed. Please do not skip doses or stop giving the medication. If you have difficulty giving doses consult your veterinarian or pharmacist who can offer administration techniques or change the dosage form to a type of medication that may be more acceptable to you and your animal.

- If you miss a dose of this medication you should give it as soon as you remember it, but if it is within a few hours of the regularly scheduled dose, wait and give it at the regular time. Do not double a dose as this can be toxic to your pet.
- Some other drugs can interact with this medication so tell your veterinarian about any drugs or foods that you currently give your animal. Do not give new foods or medications without first asking your veterinarian.
- **Dogs and Cats**: Dogs and cats usually receive vitamin E from one to three times daily with a fatty food.
- **Horses**: Horses receive vitamin E orally once daily to assist in treatment of EPM.

What Other Information Is Important About This Medication?

- Vitamin E should be stored in a tight, light resistant, childproof container away from all children and other household pets.
- Vitamin E can be purchased over the counter without a prescription.

VETERINARY DRUG HANDBOOK-Client Information Edition
Permission to photocopy for individual clients granted by Gigi Davidson and Donald C. Plumb © 2003

Warfarin

Coumadin® is another name for this medication.

How Is This Medication Useful?

- Warfarin is a blood thinner used to prevent the formation of blood clots in animals with circulation problems.

Are There Conditions or Times When Its Use Might Cause More Harm Than Good?

- Because warfarin stops the clotting of blood, it should not be used in animals with bleeding problems (*e.g.*, stomach ulcers, broken blood vessels) or that are aboute to undergo surgery.
- It should not be used in animals that are already anemic due to the increased risk for loss of blood.
- It should be used very cautiously in working animals or performance horses as the risk of uncontrollable bleeding from cuts and bruises is high.
- Warfarin should not be used in pregnant animals as it causes birth defects.
- Warfarin should not be used in animals with liver problems as it may build up in the body and cause uncontrolled bleeding.
- Warfarin affects and is affected by many different drugs and can cause fatal bleeding problems. You should tell your veterinarian about any drugs that your animal is taking.
- If your animal has any of the above conditions, talk to your veterinarian about the potential risks of using the medication versus the benefits that it might have.

What Side Effects Can Be Seen With Its Use?

- Because warfarin stops clotting, it may cause nosebleeds, bruising and other bleeding problems that can lead to anemia.

How Should It Be Given?

- Warfarin should be given orally once daily.
- The active drug in commercially available warfarin tablets may be unevenly distributed. If your veterinarian prescribes ½ or ¼ tablets, then you should crush the whole tablet, mix up the powder and then give ½ or ¼ of the powder. It may be better to have your pharmacist compound capsules of the exact dose or formulate a liquid to achieve the correct dose.

- The successful outcome of your animal's treatment with this medication depends upon your commitment and ability to administer it exactly as the veterinarian has prescribed. Please do not skip doses or stop giving the medication. If you have difficulty giving doses consult your veterinarian or pharmacist who can offer administration techniques or change the dosage form to a type of medication that may be more acceptable to you and your animal.
- If you miss a dose of this medication you should give it as soon as you remember it, but if it is within a few hours of the regularly scheduled dose, wait and give it at the regular time. Do not double a dose as this can be toxic to your pet.
- Some other drugs can interact with this medication so tell your veterinarian about any drugs or foods that you currently give your animal. Do not give new foods or medications without first asking your veterinarian.
- **Dogs and Cats**: Dogs and cats usually receive warfarin orally once daily and should be checked weekly for the first month and then monthly while on the medication.
- **Horses**: Warfarin is not usually given to horses, but can be given orally once daily. It is a Class 5 drug according to the Association of Racing Commissioners International (ARCI).

What Other Information Is Important About This Medication?

- Warfarin should be stored in a tight, light resistant, childproof container away from all children and other household pets.
- Your veterinarian will need to check blood clotting times periodically to make sure that your pet is not getting too much warfarin. It is very important to bring your pet back for these important visits.
- You should make sure that you pet does not cut itself or fight with other animals while on warfarin as it could suffer uncontrollable bleeding.

Aminoglycosides Ophthalmic

Gentocin® and Garamycin® (gentamicin), and Tobrex® (tobramycin) are other names for this medication.

How Is This Medication Useful?

- Aminoglycosides are strong antibiotics that are used to treat bacterial infections of the clear part of the eye (cornea). They are mostly used to treat cats with bacterial eye diseases.

Are There Conditions or Times When Its Use Might Cause More Harm Than Good?

- Aminoglycosides must not be used in any animals that will be used for human food.
- If your animal has any of the above conditions, talk to your veterinarian about the potential risks of using the medication versus the benefits that it might have.

What Side Effects Can Be Seen With Its Use?

- The medication may cause the eye to sting a bit when first put in the eye.
- Ointments will blur your animal's vision for a few minutes after administration. You should watch it for a short time to make sure it does not bump into things and injure itself.
- Side effects from eye use of aminoglycosides are rare, but when used by injection, aminoglycosides can cause damage to the kidneys and ears.
- Some animals will experience swelling of the lids and itching after use.
- One aminoglycoside, neomycin, is a part of triple antibiotic ophthalmic medication. This combination of antibiotics can cause a fatal allergic reaction in cats. If your cat has swelling of the face or itching or looks like it is having difficulty breathing, you should take your cat to the closest veterinary clinic immediately.
- If your cat's eye looks worse after you start the medication, you should call your veterinarian.

How Should It Be Given?

- Eye drops may be used every 2-6 hours and ointments every 8-12 depending on the condition that your veterinarian is treating.
- If you are giving more than one medication, you should allow 5 minutes between medications to allow the medication to work and to not be washed out by the next medication.

- Medication should be applied in the lower eyelid sac (conjunctival sac) without touching the tip of the dropper or tube to the eye as this will contaminate the medication. Do not touch the dropper or tube tip with your fingers as this will also contaminate the medication.
- The successful outcome of your animal's treatment with this medication depends upon your commitment and ability to administer it exactly as the veterinarian has prescribed. Please do not skip doses or stop giving the medication. If you have difficulty giving doses consult your veterinarian or pharmacist who can offer administration techniques or change the dosage form to a type of medication that may be more acceptable to you and your animal.
- If you miss a dose of this medication you should give it as soon as you remember it, but if it is within a few hours of the regularly scheduled dose, wait and give it at the regular time. Do not double a dose as this can be toxic to your pet.
- Some other drugs can interact with this medication so tell your veterinarian about any drugs or foods that you currently give your animal. Do not give new foods or medications without first asking your veterinarian.
- You should always wash your hands after applying this medication to your pet's eyes.
- **Dogs and Cats**: Aminoglycosides are usually administered as a drop three to six times daily. They may also be administered as an ointment two to three times daily.
- **Horses**: Horses will usually receive aminoglycosides as a solution administered through an eye catheter (subpalpebral lavage system) every one to four hours.

What Other Information Is Important About This Medication?

- Aminoglycosides should be stored in a tight, light resistant, childproof container away from all children and other household pets.
- Your pet's eye should start to look better in 48 hours. If the eye looks the same or gets worse, you should contact your veterinarian for advice.

VETERINARY DRUG HANDBOOK-Client Information Edition
Permission to photocopy for individual clients granted by Gigi Davidson and Donald C. Plumb © 2003

Atropine Sulfate Ophthalmic

Atrophate® is another name for this medication.

How Is This Medication Useful?

- Atropine sulfate is used in the eye to dilate the pupil. This effect is useful in reducing pain after cataract surgery or eye injury and is also useful in treating glaucoma.

Are There Conditions or Times When Its Use Might Cause More Harm Than Good?

- Condition may worsen with atropine use in dogs with primary glaucoma.
- Using atropine in the eye more frequently than prescribed can result in serious problems such as colic in horses and a dangerous increase in body temperature in other animals.
- Atropine toxicity may also cause some changes in heart rate and rhythm and may cause your pet to be unable to urinate.
- If your animal has any of the above conditions, talk to your veterinarian about the potential risks of using the medication versus the benefits that it might have.

What Side Effects Can Be Seen With Its Use?

- Because atropine dilates the pupil, animals will be very sensitive to sunlight and should be kept out of bright light while receiving this drug.
- Most animals will salivate when atropine drops get into their mouth.
- Too much atropine can result in dry mouth, constipation and vomiting.

How Should It Be Given?

- The successful outcome of your animal's treatment with this medication depends upon your commitment and ability to administer it exactly as the veterinarian has prescribed. Please do not skip doses or stop giving the medication. If you have difficulty giving doses consult your veterinarian or pharmacist who can offer administration techniques or change the dosage form to a type of medication that may be more acceptable to you and your animal.

- If you miss a dose of this medication you should give it as soon as you remember it, but if it is within a few hours of the regularly scheduled dose, wait and give it at the regular time. Do not double a dose as this can be toxic to your pet.
- Some other drugs can interact with this medication so tell your veterinarian about any drugs or foods that you currently give your animal. Do not give new foods or medications without first asking your veterinarian.
- You should always wash your hands after applying this medication to your pet's eyes as it can get into your eyes and cause dilation of the pupil.
- **Dogs and Cats**: Atropine sulfate has a very long duration of action and is usually administered no more than once daily in dogs and cats.
- **Horses**: Horses will usually receive atropine sulfate as an ointment once daily or as a solution administered through an eye catheter (subpalpebral lavage system).

What Other Information Is Important About This Medication?

- Atropine sulfate should be stored in a tight, light resistant, childproof container away from all children and other household pets.

Chloramphenicol Ophthalmic

Bemacol®, Chlorbiotic® and Chloricol® are other names for this medication.

How Is This Medication Useful?

- Chloramphenicol is an antibiotic that can penetrate the cornea (clear part of the eye) and reach inside the eye to treat infections. It is mostly used to treat cats with bacterial eye diseases.

Are There Conditions or Times When Its Use Might Cause More Harm Than Good?

- Some humans have a fatal allergic reaction to chloramphenicol. This reaction does not occur in animals, but you should always wear gloves when applying chloramphenicol and wash hands afterwards.
- Chloramphenicol must not be used in any animals that will be used for human food.
- If your animal has any of the above conditions, talk to your veterinarian about the potential risks of using the medication versus the benefits that it might have.

What Side Effects Can Be Seen With Its Use?

- The medication may cause the eye to sting a bit when first put in the eye.
- Ointments will blur your animal's vision for a few minutes after administration. You should watch it for a short time to make sure it does not bump into things and injure itself.
- Side effects from chloramphenicol administered in the eye are rare, but prolonged or excessive use of chloramphenicol can cause the same side effects as when chloramphenicol is swallowed.
- Because chloramphenicol can cause blood problems, it should not be used in animals who are already experiencing anemias or bleeding abnormalities.
- Chloramphenicol must be eliminated from the body by the liver and should not be used in patients who have liver failure. If it must be used, then a reduced dose is required but then the risk of not curing the infection is a possibility.
- Chloramphenicol should be used with extreme caution, if at all, in baby animals. This drug can cause the blood vessels to fail to properly circulate blood resulting in lack of oxygen to vital organs. This drug is particularly dangerous when used in kittens.
- Because chloramphenicol is secreted in the milk, it should not be given to nursing mothers.
- Chloramphenicol should also not be used in breeding animals, and should not be used in pregnancy due to adverse effects on the bone marrow of the fetus.

How Should It Be Given?

- Eye drops may be used every 2-6 hours and ointments every 8-12 depending on the condition that your veterinarian is treating.
- If you are giving more than one medication, you should allow 5 minutes between medications to allow the medication to work and to not be washed out by the next medication.
- Medication should be applied in the lower eyelid sac (conjunctival sac) without touching the tip of the dropper or tube to the eye as this will contaminate the medication. Do not touch the dropper or tube tip with your fingers as this will also contaminate the medication.
- The successful outcome of your animal's treatment with this medication depends upon your commitment and ability to administer it exactly as the veterinarian has prescribed. Please do not skip doses or stop giving the medication. If you have difficulty giving doses consult your veterinarian or pharmacist who can offer administration techniques or change the dosage form to a type of medication that may be more acceptable to you and your animal.
- If you miss a dose of this medication you should give it as soon as you remember it, but if it is within a few hours of the regularly scheduled dose, wait and give it at the regular time. Do not double a dose as this can be toxic to your pet.
- Some other drugs can interact with this medication so tell your veterinarian about any drugs or foods that you currently give your animal. Do not give new foods or medications without first asking your veterinarian.
- You should always wash your hands after applying this medication to your pet's eyes as it can get into your eyes and cause harm or death if you are allergic to chloramphenicol.
- **Dogs and Cats:** Chloramphenicol is usually administered as an ointment three times daily.
- **Horses:** Horses will usually receive chloramphenicol as an ointment two to three times daily or as a solution administered through an eye catheter (subpalpebral lavage system).

What Other Information Is Important About This Medication?

- Chloramphenicol should be stored in a tight, light resistant, childproof container away from all children and other household pets.
- Your pet's eye should start to look better in 48 hours. If the eye looks the same or gets worse, you should contact your veterinarian for advice.

Corticosteroids Ophthalmic

Decadron®, Pred Forte® and Econopred® are other names for this medication.

How Is This Medication Useful?

- Corticosteroids are used in the eye to stop inflammation. The ones most commonly used in the eye are prednisolone and dexamethasone. They should not be used in animals with an infected eye ulcer.

Are There Conditions or Times When Its Use Might Cause More Harm Than Good?

- Corticosteroids should not be used in animals that are allergic to them or to drugs like them.
- Corticosteroids should not be used in the presence of ulcers infected with bacteria or fungus.
- Corticosteroids may cause problems in pets with diabetes or Cushing's disease.

What Side Effects Can Be Seen With Its Use?

- Corticosteroids have few known side effects when used in the eye. You should not use more than prescribed and you should not get the drops on the animals face or in its mouth. You should prevent your pet from licking the drops off.

How Should It Be Given?

- Corticosteroids are used once or twice daily for inflammation of the eye. Corticosteroid drops should be shaken well before use.
- The successful outcome of your animal's treatment with this medication depends upon your commitment and ability to administer it exactly as the veterinarian has prescribed. Please do not skip doses or stop giving the medication. If you have difficulty giving doses consult your veterinarian or pharmacist who can offer administration techniques or change the dosage form to a type of medication that may be more acceptable to you and your animal.
- If you miss a dose of this medication you should give it as soon as you remember it, but if it is within a few hours of the regularly scheduled dose, wait and give it at the regular time. Do not double a dose as this can be toxic to your pet.

- Some other drugs can interact with this medication so tell your veterinarian about any drugs or foods that you currently give your animal. Do not give new foods or medications without first asking your veterinarian.
- You should always wash your hands after applying this medication to your pet's eyes as it can get into your eyes and cause dilation of the pupil.
- **Dogs and Cats**: Corticosteroids are usually administered four times daily for inflammation in dogs and cats.
- **Horses**: Horses may receive corticosteroids once or twice daily as a drop or an ointment.

What Other Information Is Important About This Medication?

- Corticosteroids should be stored in a tight, light resistant, childproof container away from all children and other household pets.
- Corticosteroid drops should be shaken well before use.

Cyclosporine Ophthalmic

Optimune® is another name for this medication.

How Is This Medication Useful?

- Cyclosporine is a strong immune-suppressing medication that is used to treat dry eye in dogs and may also be useful in treating other inflammatory diseases of the eye such as pannus in German Shepherds or chronic uveitis (Moon blindness) in horses. It does not cure these conditions and must be given for the rest of the animal's life.

Are There Conditions or Times When Its Use Might Cause More Harm Than Good?

- Cyclosporine may prevent healing of ulcers of the clear part of the eye (cornea) and should be used with caution in animals who have an eye ulcer.
- Some dogs do not respond to the ointment form of the drug and must receive the drops. Cyclosporine drops will have to be specially formulated by a compounding pharmacist as they are not commercially available.
- It can cause weakening of the human immune system, so you should wear gloves or wash hands after applying this medication to your pet's eye.

What Side Effects Can Be Seen With Its Use?

- Cyclosporine has few side effects when applied to the eye.

How Should It Be Given?

- Cyclosporine ointment is used every 12 hours for the rest of the pet's life.
- If you are giving more than one eye medication, you should allow 5 minutes between medications to allow the medication to work and to not be washed out by the next medication.
- Medication should be applied in the lower eyelid sac (conjunctival sac) without touching the tip of the dropper or tube to the eye as this will contaminate the medication. Do not touch the dropper or tube tip with your fingers as this will also contaminate the medication.

- The successful outcome of your animal's treatment with this medication depends upon your commitment and ability to administer it exactly as the veterinarian has prescribed. Please do not skip doses or stop giving the medication. If you have difficulty giving doses consult your veterinarian or pharmacist who can offer administration techniques or change the dosage form to a type of medication that may be more acceptable to you and your animal.
- If you miss a dose of this medication you should give it as soon as you remember it, but if it is within a few hours of the regularly scheduled dose, wait and give it at the regular time. Do not double a dose as this can be toxic to your pet.
- Some other drugs can interact with this medication so tell your veterinarian about any drugs or foods that you currently give your animal. Do not give new foods or medications without first asking your veterinarian.
- You should always wash your hands after applying this medication to your pet's eyes.
- **Dogs and Cats**: Cyclosporine is usually administered twice daily as an ointment for the rest of the pet's life.
- **Horses**: Horses will usually receive cyclosporine as an ointment administered once or twice daily. Some veterinary ophthalmologists may implant a bead of cyclosporine inside your horse's eye instead of having you use ointment twice daily.

What Other Information Is Important About This Medication?

- Cyclosporine should be stored in a tight, light resistant, childproof container away from all children and other household pets. It should not be refrigerated.
- Cyclosporine drops will have to be specially formulated by a compounding pharmacist and may be expensive. You should call for refills well ahead of the time you need them to ensure that the pharmacist has had time to make this eye drop.
- Your horse's eye(s) should start to look better in 48 hours. If the eye looks the same or gets worse, you should contact your veterinarian for advice.

VETERINARY DRUG HANDBOOK-Client Information Edition
Permission to photocopy for individual clients granted by Gigi Davidson and Donald C. Plumb © 2003

Dorzolamide Ophthalmic

Trusopt® is another name for this medication.

How Is This Medication Useful?

- Dorzolamide is used in the eye to reduce the pressure caused by glaucoma. It is most often used in the "good" eye to prevent glaucoma formation after glaucoma has been diagnosed in the other eye.

Are There Conditions or Times When Its Use Might Cause More Harm Than Good?

- Dorzolamide given topically has no known contraindications.

What Side Effects Can Be Seen With Its Use?

- Dorzolamide stings when placed in the eye. It does not make the pupil become smaller like other glaucoma drugs.

How Should It Be Given?

- Dorzolamide should be used three times daily.
- The successful outcome of your animal's treatment with this medication depends upon your commitment and ability to administer it exactly as the veterinarian has prescribed. Please do not skip doses or stop giving the medication. If you have difficulty giving doses consult your veterinarian or pharmacist who can offer administration techniques or change the dosage form to a type of medication that may be more acceptable to you and your animal.

- If you miss a dose of this medication you should give it as soon as you remember it, but if it is within a few hours of the regularly scheduled dose, wait and give it at the regular time. Do not double a dose as this can be toxic to your pet.
- Some other drugs can interact with this medication so tell your veterinarian about any drugs or foods that you currently give your animal. Do not give new foods or medications without first asking your veterinarian.
- You should always wash your hands after applying this medication to your pet's eyes as it can get into your eyes and cause dilation of the pupil.
- **Dogs and Cats**: Dorzolamide is usually administered three times daily in dogs and cats.
- **Horses**: Horses do not usually receive dorzolamide.

What Other Information Is Important About This Medication?

- Dorzolamide should be stored in a tight, light resistant, childproof container away from all children and other household pets.

Flurbiprofen Ophthalmic

Ocufen® is another name for this medication.

How Is This Medication Useful?

- Flurbiprofen is used in the eye to stop inflammation in the eye.

Are There Conditions or Times When Its Use Might Cause More Harm Than Good?

- Flurbiprofen should not be used in animals that are allergic to it or to drugs like it.
- Flurbiprofen may increase the pressure in the eye and should not be used in patients with glaucoma.
- It should not be used in animals that have an infected eye ulcer as it may get worse.
- If your animal has any of the above conditions, talk to your veterinarian about the potential risks of using the medication versus the benefits that it might have.

What Side Effects Can Be Seen With Its Use?

- Flurbiprofen will make the pupil get smaller.
- Flurbiprofen makes the pressure go up in the eye.

How Should It Be Given?

- Flurbiprofen is used once or twice daily for inflammation of the eye.
- The successful outcome of your animal's treatment with this medication depends upon your commitment and ability to administer it exactly as the veterinarian has prescribed. Please do not skip doses or stop giving the medication. If you have difficulty giving doses consult your veterinarian or pharmacist who can offer administration techniques or change the dosage form to a type of medication that may be more acceptable to you and your animal.

- If you miss a dose of this medication you should give it as soon as you remember it, but if it is within a few hours of the regularly scheduled dose, wait and give it at the regular time. Do not double a dose as this can be toxic to your pet.
- Some other drugs can interact with this medication so tell your veterinarian about any drugs or foods that you currently give your animal. Do not give new foods or medications without first asking your veterinarian.
- You should always wash your hands after applying this medication to your pet's eyes as it can get into your eyes and cause dilation of the pupil.
- **Dogs and Cats**: Flurbiprofen is usually administered once or twice daily for inflammation in dogs and cats.
- **Horses**: Horses do not usually receive flurbiprofen.

What Other Information Is Important About This Medication?

- Flurbiprofen should be stored in a tight, light resistant, childproof container away from all children and other household pets.

Idoxuridine Ophthalmic

Stoxil® is another name for this medication.

How Is This Medication Useful?

- Idoxuridine is an antiviral medication that is used to treat viral infections of the eye. It is mostly used to treat cats with viral eye diseases such as herpes.
- Idoxuridine is no longer available as a commercially available drug product and will have to be compounded into an eye drop by a compounding pharmacist. It may be expensive, but is not as expensive as trifluridine, another anti-viral eye drop.

Are There Conditions or Times When Its Use Might Cause More Harm Than Good?

- Since herpes infection is triggered by stress, the frequent administration of this drug which also stings, may cause worsening of the condition.
- If your animal does not appear to be getting better, talk to your veterinarian about the potential risks of using the medication versus the benefits that it might have.

What Side Effects Can Be Seen With Its Use?

- The medication may cause the eye to sting a bit when first put in the eye.
- Ointments will blur your animal's vision for a few minutes after administration. You should watch it for a short time to make sure it does not bump into things and injure itself.

How Should It Be Given?

- Eye drops may be used every 2-6 hours depending on the condition that your veterinarian is treating.
- If you are giving more than one medication, you should allow 5 minutes between medications to allow the medication to work and to not be washed out by the next medication.

- Medication should be applied in the lower eyelid sac (conjunctival sac) without touching the tip of the dropper or tube to the eye as this will contaminate the medication. Do not touch the dropper or tube tip with your fingers as this will also contaminate the medication.
- The successful outcome of your animal's treatment with this medication depends upon your commitment and ability to administer it exactly as the veterinarian has prescribed. Please do not skip doses or stop giving the medication. If you have difficulty giving doses consult your veterinarian or pharmacist who can offer administration techniques or change the dosage form to a type of medication that may be more acceptable to you and your animal.
- If you miss a dose of this medication you should give it as soon as you remember it, but if it is within a few hours of the regularly scheduled dose, wait and give it at the regular time. Do not double a dose as this can be toxic to your pet.
- Some other drugs can interact with this medication so tell your veterinarian about any drugs or foods that you currently give your animal. Do not give new foods or medications without first asking your veterinarian.
- You should always wash your hands after applying this medication to your pet's eyes.
- **Dogs and Cats**: Idoxuridine is not usually given to dogs but is usually administered as a drop three to six times daily for cats.
- **Horses**: Horses do not usually receive this medication.
-

What Other Information Is Important About This Medication?

- Idoxuridine should be stored in a tight, light resistant, childproof container in the refrigerator away from all children and other household pets.
- Your pet's eye should start to look better in 48 hours. If the eye looks the same or gets worse, you should contact your veterinarian for advice.

Itraconazole in DMSO Ophthalmic

Sporonox® is another name for this medication.

How Is This Medication Useful?

- Itraconazole is a strong antifungal medication that is used to treat fungus infections of the clear part (cornea) of the eyes. This condition usually occurs in horses and treatment usually lasts at least 4-6 weeks.
- Itraconazole is no longer available as a commercially available ophthalmic drug and will have to be compounded into an eye ointment by a compounding pharmacist. It may be expensive but is not as expensive as natamycin, another antifungal eye drop.

Are There Conditions or Times When Its Use Might Cause More Harm Than Good?

- Itraconazole is usually administered as an ointment directly to the eye sac as it is too thick to be administered as a liquid.
- This ointment contains a chemical called DMSO which may be hazardous to some humans. You should wear gloves while applying this ointment and wash hands afterwards.

What Side Effects Can Be Seen With Its Use?

- Once the medication starts killing off the fungus, the eye will at first become swollen and cloudy. This is a good sign that the fungus are dying. If this persists after 48 hours you should call your veterinarian.

How Should It Be Given?

- Itraconazole ointment may be used every 1-2 hours during the first few days of treatment and then four to six times daily for 4-6 weeks afterwards.
- If you are giving more than one medication, you should allow 5 minutes between medications to allow the medication to work and to not be washed out by the next medication.
- Medication should be applied in the lower eyelid sac (conjunctival sac) without touching the tip of the dropper or tube to the eye as this will contaminate the medication. Do not touch the dropper or tube tip with your fingers as this will also contaminate the medication.

- The successful outcome of your animal's treatment with this medication depends upon your commitment and ability to administer it exactly as the veterinarian has prescribed. Please do not skip doses or stop giving the medication. If you have difficulty giving doses consult your veterinarian or pharmacist who can offer administration techniques or change the dosage form to a type of medication that may be more acceptable to you and your animal.
- If you miss a dose of this medication you should give it as soon as you remember it, but if it is within a few hours of the regularly scheduled dose, wait and give it at the regular time. Do not double a dose as this can be toxic to your pet.
- Some other drugs can interact with this medication so tell your veterinarian about any drugs or foods that you currently give your animal. Do not give new foods or medications without first asking your veterinarian.
- You should always wash your hands after applying this medication to your pet's eyes.
- **Dogs and Cats**: Itraconazole is not usually administered to dogs or cats.
- **Horses**: Horses will usually receive itraconazole as an ointment administered every two to three hours for the first few days and then every 4-6 hours afterwards for 4-6 weeks.

What Other Information Is Important About This Medication?

- Itraconazole should be stored in a tight, light resistant, childproof container away from all children and other household pets.
- Itraconazole has to be specially formulated by a compounding pharmacist and may be expensive. You should call for refills well ahead of the time you need them to ensure that the pharmacist has had time to make this ointment.
- Your horse's eye should start to look better in 48 hours. If the eye looks the same or gets worse, you should contact your veterinarian for advice.

Ketorolac Ophthalmic

Acular® is another name for this medication.

How Is This Medication Useful?

- Ketorolac is used in the eye to stop inflammation.

Are There Conditions or Times When Its Use Might Cause More Harm Than Good?

- Ketorolac should not be used in animals that are allergic to it or to drugs like it.

What Side Effects Can Be Seen With Its Use?

- Ketorolac has few known side effects. Cats should not be allowed to groom ketorolac off of their eyes as it can cause problems (bleeding and kidney damage) in cats when swallowed.

How Should It Be Given?

- Ketorolac is used once or twice daily for inflammation of the eye.
- The successful outcome of your animal's treatment with this medication depends upon your commitment and ability to administer it exactly as the veterinarian has prescribed. Please do not skip doses or stop giving the medication. If you have difficulty giving doses consult your veterinarian or pharmacist who can offer administration techniques or change the dosage form to a type of medication that may be more acceptable to you and your animal.
- If you miss a dose of this medication you should give it as soon as you remember it, but if it is within a few hours of the regularly scheduled dose, wait and give it at the regular time. Do not double a dose as this can be toxic to your pet.

- Some other drugs can interact with this medication so tell your veterinarian about any drugs or foods that you currently give your animal. Do not give new foods or medications without first asking your veterinarian.
- You should always wash your hands after applying this medication to your pet's eyes as it can get into your eyes and cause dilation of the pupil.
- **Dogs and Cats**: Ketorolac is usually administered four times daily for inflammation in dogs and cats.
- **Horses**: Horses do not usually receive ketorolac.

What Other Information Is Important About This Medication?

- Ketorolac should be stored in a tight, light resistant, childproof container away from all children and other household pets.

Latanaprost Ophthalmic

Xalatan® is another name for this medication.

How Is This Medication Useful?
- Latanaprost is used in the eye to reduce the pressure caused by glaucoma.

Are There Conditions or Times When Its Use Might Cause More Harm Than Good?
- Latanaprost might not work as well if you use it more than twice daily.
- It does not seem to work well to manage glaucoma in cats.
- If your animal has any of the above conditions, talk to your veterinarian about the potential risks of using the medication versus the benefits that it might have.

What Side Effects Can Be Seen With Its Use?
- Latanaprost may sting when placed in the eye.
- Animals with light colored irises may develop brown irises.
- Latanaprost will cause the pupil (black part) of the eye to become much smaller. Your veterinarian may ask your pharmacist to dilute the latanaprost to half-strength to reduce this effect.

How Should It Be Given?
- Latanaprost is usually started at once daily but may be increased to twice daily. It should not be used more than twice daily or it may stop working.
- Latanaprost is a prostaglandin drug that can cause pregnant women to miscarry. If you are pregnant, you should wear gloves or have someone else give the eye drops.
- The successful outcome of your animal's treatment with this medication depends upon your commitment and ability to administer it exactly as the veterinarian has prescribed. Please do not skip doses or stop giving the medication. If you have difficulty giving doses consult your veterinarian or pharmacist who can offer administration techniques or change the dosage form to a type of medication that may be more acceptable to you and your animal.

- If you miss a dose of this medication you should give it as soon as you remember it, but if it is within a few hours of the regularly scheduled dose, wait and give it at the regular time. Do not double a dose as this can be toxic to your pet.
- Some other drugs can interact with this medication so tell your veterinarian about any drugs or foods that you currently give your animal. Do not give new foods or medications without first asking your veterinarian.
- You should always wash your hands after applying this medication to your pet's eyes as it can get into your eyes and cause dilation of the pupil.
- **Dogs and Cats**: Latanaprost is usually administered three times daily in dogs and cats.
- **Horses**: Horses do not usually receive latanaprost.

What Other Information Is Important About This Medication?
- Latanaprost should be stored in a tight, light resistant, childproof container in the refrigerator away from all children and other household pets.

Miconazole Ophthalmic

Monistat® is another name for this medication.

How Is This Medication Useful?

- Miconazole is a strong antifungal medication that is used to treat fungus infections of the clear part (cornea) of the eyes. This condition usually occurs in horses and treatment usually lasts at least 4-6 weeks.
- Miconazole is no longer available as a commercially available drug and will have to be compounded into an eye drop by a compounding pharmacist. It may be expensive but is not as expensive as natamycin, another anti-fungal eye drop.

Are There Conditions or Times When Its Use Might Cause More Harm Than Good?

- Miconazole is usually administered through a special eye catheter (subpalpebral lavage system) that your veterinarian has placed under your horse's skin. If it leaks out of the catheter into the skin around your horse's eye, it may be irritating and painful and it won't get to the eye where it needs to work. If you think that your catheter is leaking you should contact your veterinarian immediately.

What Side Effects Can Be Seen With Its Use?

- Once the medication starts killing off the fungus, the eye will at first become swollen and cloudy. This is a good sign that the fungus is dying. If this persists after 48 hours you should call your veterinarian.

How Should It Be Given?

- Eye drops may be used every 1-2 hours during the first few days of treatment and then four to six times daily for 4-6 weeks afterwards.
- If you are giving more than one medication, you should allow 5 minutes between medications to allow the medication to work and to not be washed out by the next medication. If you are placing medications through the catheter system, you should push some air, not liquid, through the tubing between drugs to push the drops to the eye.

- Medication should be applied in the lower eyelid sac (conjunctival sac) without touching the tip of the dropper or tube to the eye as this will contaminate the medication. Do not touch the dropper or tube tip with your fingers as this will also contaminate the medication.
- The successful outcome of your animal's treatment with this medication depends upon your commitment and ability to administer it exactly as the veterinarian has prescribed. Please do not skip doses or stop giving the medication. If you have difficulty giving doses consult your veterinarian or pharmacist who can offer administration techniques or change the dosage form to a type of medication that may be more acceptable to you and your animal.
- If you miss a dose of this medication you should give it as soon as you remember it, but if it is within a few hours of the regularly scheduled dose, wait and give it at the regular time. Do not double a dose as this can be toxic to your pet.
- Some other drugs can interact with this medication so tell your veterinarian about any drugs or foods that you currently give your animal. Do not give new foods or medications without first asking your veterinarian.
- You should always wash your hands after applying this medication to your pet's eyes.
- **Dogs and Cats**: Miconazole is not usually administered to dogs or cats.
- **Horses**: Horses will usually receive miconazole as a solution administered through an eye catheter (subpalpebral lavage system) every one to two hours for the first few days and then every 4-6 hours afterwards for 4-6 weeks.

What Other Information Is Important About This Medication?

- Miconazole should be stored in a tight, light resistant, childproof container away from all children and other household pets.
- Miconazole has to be specially formulated by a compounding pharmacist and may be expensive. You should call for refills well before you need them to ensure that the pharmacist has had time to prepare this medication.
- Your horse's eye should start to look better in 48 hours. If the eye looks the same or gets worse, you should contact your veterinarian for advice.

Natamycin Ophthalmic

Natacyn® is another name for this medication.

How Is This Medication Useful?

- Natamycin is a strong antifungal medication that is used to treat fungus infections of the clear part (cornea) of the eyes. This condition usually occurs in horses and treatment usually lasts at least 4-6 weeks.

Are There Conditions or Times When Its Use Might Cause More Harm Than Good?

- Natamycin is a thick white liquid that may clog the special eye catheter (subpalpebral lavage system) that your veterinarian has placed under your horse's skin. If it leaks out of the catheter into the skin around your horse's eye, it will be very painful. Your veterinarian may want you to put the drops directly into the sac of the eye and not use the catheter.

What Side Effects Can Be Seen With Its Use?

- This medication will likely cause stinging when placed in the eye.
- Once the medication starts killing off the fungus, the eye will at first become swollen and cloudy. This is a good sign that the fungus is dying. If this persists after 48 hours you should call your veterinarian.
- Natamycin is thick and milky and will blur your horse's vision for a few minutes after administration. You should watch it for a short time to make sure it does not bump into things and injure itself or its eye.

How Should It Be Given?

- Eye drops may be used every 1-2 hours during the first few days of treatment and then four to six times daily for 4-6 weeks afterwards. Natamycin should be shaken well before using.
- If you are giving more than one medication, you should allow 5 minutes between medications to allow the medication to work and to not be washed out by the next medication. If you are placing medications through the catheter system, you should push some air, not liquid, through the tubing between drugs to push the drops to the eye.

- Medication should be applied in the lower eyelid sac (conjunctival sac) without touching the tip of the dropper or tube to the eye as this will contaminate the medication. Do not touch the dropper or tube tip with your fingers as this will also contaminate the medication.
- The successful outcome of your animal's treatment with this medication depends upon your commitment and ability to administer it exactly as the veterinarian has prescribed. Please do not skip doses or stop giving the medication. If you have difficulty giving doses consult your veterinarian or pharmacist who can offer administration techniques or change the dosage form to a type of medication that may be more acceptable to you and your animal.
- If you miss a dose of this medication you should give it as soon as you remember it, but if it is within a few hours of the regularly scheduled dose, wait and give it at the regular time. Do not double a dose as this can be toxic to your pet.
- Some other drugs can interact with this medication so tell your veterinarian about any drugs or foods that you currently give your animal. Do not give new foods or medications without first asking your veterinarian.
- You should always wash your hands after applying this medication to your pet's eyes.
- **Dogs and Cats**: Natamycin is not usually administered to dogs or cats.
- **Horses**: Horses will usually receive natamycin as a solution administered through an eye catheter (subpalpebral lavage system) every one to two hours for the first few days and then every 4-6 hours afterwards for 4-6 weeks.

What Other Information Is Important About This Medication?

- Natamycin should be stored in a tight, light resistant, childproof container away from all children and other household pets. It should be shaken well before use.
- Natamycin is very expensive.
- Your horse's eye should start to look better in 48 hours. If the eye looks the same or gets worse, you should contact your veterinarian for advice.

Oxytetracycline Ophthalmic

Terramycin® is another name for this medication.

How Is This Medication Useful?

• Oxytetracycline is a strong antibiotic that is used to treat bacterial infections of the clear part of the eye (cornea) and the pink parts around the eyelids (conjunctiva). It is mostly used to treat cats with bacterial eye diseases or to treat pink eye.

Are There Conditions or Times When Its Use Might Cause More Harm Than Good?

• There are very few side effects associated with oxytetracyline use in the eye. Some cats will be allergic to one of the other ingredients (polymyxin) in Terramycin®. If your cat's eye looks worse after you start the medication, you should call your veterinarian.

What Side Effects Can Be Seen With Its Use?

• The medication may cause the eye to sting a bit when first put in the eye.
• Ointments will blur your animal's vision for a few minutes after administration. You should watch it for a short time to make sure it does not bump into things and injure itself.
• Side effects from eye use of oxytetracycline are rare, but when used orally or by injection, oxytetracycline can cause discoloration of the teeth of young animals and can increase the risk of severe sunburn while in direct sunlight.
• Some animals will experience swelling of the lids and itching after use. You should call your veterinarian if this happens.

How Should It Be Given?

• Eye drops may be used every 2-6 hours and ointments every 8-12 depending on the condition that your veterinarian is treating.
• If you are giving more than one medication, you should allow 5 minutes between medications to allow the medication to work and to not be washed out by the next medication.
• Medication should be applied in the lower eyelid sac (conjunctival sac) without touching the tip of the dropper or tube to the eye as this will contaminate the medication. Do not touch the dropper or tube tip with your fingers as this will also contaminate the medication.

• The successful outcome of your animal's treatment with this medication depends upon your commitment and ability to administer it exactly as the veterinarian has prescribed. Please do not skip doses or stop giving the medication. If you have difficulty giving doses consult your veterinarian or pharmacist who can offer administration techniques or change the dosage form to a type of medication that may be more acceptable to you and your animal.
• If you miss a dose of this medication you should give it as soon as you remember it, but if it is within a few hours of the regularly scheduled dose, wait and give it at the regular time. Do not double a dose as this can be toxic to your pet.
• Some other drugs can interact with this medication so tell your veterinarian about any drugs or foods that you currently give your animal. Do not give new foods or medications without first asking your veterinarian.
• You should always wash your hands after applying this medication to your pet's eyes.
• **Dogs and Cats**: Oxytetracycline are usually administered as an ointment three to four times daily.
• **Horses**: Horses will usually receive oxytetracycline as an ointment once or twice daily.

What Other Information Is Important About This Medication?

• Oxytetracycline should be stored in a tight, light resistant, childproof container away from all children and other household pets.
• Your pet's eye should start to look better in 48 hours. If the eye looks the same or gets worse, you should contact your veterinarian for advice.

Fluoroquinolones Ophthalmic

Ciloxan® (ciprofloxacin), Chibroxin® (norfloxacin), and Ocuflox® (Ofloxacin) are other names for these medications.

How Is This Medication Useful?

- Fluoroquinolones are strong antibiotics that are used to treat bacterial infections of the clear part of the eye (cornea). They are mostly used to treat cats with bacterial eye infections.

Are There Conditions or Times When Its Use Might Cause More Harm Than Good?

- Fluoroquinolones must not be used in any animals that will be used for human food.
- If your animal has any of the above conditions, talk to your veterinarian about the potential risks of using the medication versus the benefits that it might have.

What Side Effects Can Be Seen With Its Use?

- The medication may cause the eye to sting a bit when first put in the eye.
- Ointments will blur your animal's vision for a few minutes after administration. You should watch it for a short time to make sure it does not bump into things and injure itself.
- Side effects from fluoroquinolones administered in the eye are rare, but prolonged or excessive use of fluoroquinolones can cause the same side effects as when fluoroquinolones are swallowed.
- Use of one fluoroquinolone, enrofloxacin, either by mouth or injection, has cause blindness in cats when used at certain doses. There have not been any reports of blindness from use of fluoroquinolones in the eye, but if your cat's pupil looks bigger than usual, you should see a veterinarian immediately.
- Use of fluoroquinolones orally and by injection have also stopped bone growth in young animals. This side effect is not likely with eye use.

How Should It Be Given?

- Eye drops may be used every 2-6 hours and ointments every 8-12 depending on the condition that your veterinarian is treating.
- If you are giving more than one medication, you should allow 5 minutes between medications to allow the medication to work and to not be washed out by the next medication. If you are placing medications through the catheter system, you should push some air, not liquid,

through the tubing between drugs to push the drops to the eye.

- Medication should be applied in the lower eyelid sac (conjunctival sac) without touching the tip of the dropper or tube to the eye as this will contaminate the medication. Do not touch the dropper or tube tip with your fingers as this will also contaminate the medication.
- The successful outcome of your animal's treatment with this medication depends upon your commitment and ability to administer it exactly as the veterinarian has prescribed. Please do not skip doses or stop giving the medication. If you have difficulty giving doses consult your veterinarian or pharmacist who can offer administration techniques or change the dosage form to a type of medication that may be more acceptable to you and your animal.
- If you miss a dose of this medication you should give it as soon as you remember it, but if it is within a few hours of the regularly scheduled dose, wait and give it at the regular time. Do not double a dose as this can be toxic to your pet.
- Some other drugs can interact with this medication so tell your veterinarian about any drugs or foods that you currently give your animal. Do not give new foods or medications without first asking your veterinarian.
- You should always wash your hands after applying this medication to your pet's eyes.
- **Dogs and Cats**: Fluoroquinolones are usually administered as a drop three to six times daily.
- **Horses**: Horses will usually receive fluoroquinolones as a solution administered through an eye catheter (subpalpebral lavage system) every one to four hours.

What Other Information Is Important About This Medication?

- Fluoroquinolones should be stored in a tight, light resistant, childproof container away from all children and other household pets.
- Your pet's eye should start to look better in 48 hours. If the eye looks the same or gets worse, you should contact your veterinarian for advice.

Timolol
Ophthalmic

Timoptic® is another name for this medication.

How Is This Medication Useful?

- Timolol is used in the eye to reduce the pressure caused by glaucoma. It is most often used in the "good" eye to prevent glaucoma formation after glaucoma has been diagnosed in the other eye.

Are There Conditions or Times When Its Use Might Cause More Harm Than Good?

- Timolol is available in 0.5% and 0.25% solutions. The 0.25% solutions do not work in animals. You should check to make sure that you have received the 0.5% solution.
- Timolol and drugs like it (beta blockers) should be used with caution in cats with asthma as it may trigger an asthma attack.
- Timolol should also be used with caution in animals that have congestive heart failure.
- If your animal has any of the above conditions, talk to your veterinarian about the potential risks of using the medication versus the benefits that it might have.

What Side Effects Can Be Seen With Its Use?

- Timolol may cause the pupil (black part) of the eye to become smaller.

How Should It Be Given?

- The successful outcome of your animal's treatment with this medication depends upon your commitment and ability to administer it exactly as the veterinarian has prescribed. Please do not skip doses or stop giving the medication. If you have difficulty giving doses consult your veterinarian or pharmacist who can offer administration techniques or change the dosage form to a type of medication that may be more acceptable to you and your animal.

- If you miss a dose of this medication you should give it as soon as you remember it, but if it is within a few hours of the regularly scheduled dose, wait and give it at the regular time. Do not double a dose as this can be toxic to your pet.
- Some other drugs can interact with this medication so tell your veterinarian about any drugs or foods that you currently give your animal. Do not give new foods or medications without first asking your veterinarian.
- You should always wash your hands after applying this medication to your pet's eyes as it can get into your eyes and cause dilation of the pupil.
- **Dogs and Cats**: Timolol is usually administered three times daily in dogs and cats.
- **Horses**: Horses do not usually receive timolol.

What Other Information Is Important About This Medication?

- Timolol should be stored in a tight, light resistant, childproof container away from all children and other household pets.

Trifluridine Ophthalmic

Viroptic® is another name for this medication.

How Is This Medication Useful?
- Trifluridine is an antiviral medication that is used to treat viral infections of the eye. It is mostly used to treat cats with viral eye diseases such as herpes.

Are There Conditions or Times When Its Use Might Cause More Harm Than Good?
- Since herpes infection is triggered by stress, the frequent administration of this drug may cause worsening of the condition.
- Trifluridine should not be used in animals who are allergic to it or have had chemical intolerance to it.
- If your animal does not appear to be getting better, talk to your veterinarian about the potential risks of using the medication versus the benefits that it might have.

What Side Effects Can Be Seen With Its Use?
- The medication may cause the eye to sting a bit when first put in the eye.
- Trifluridine may cause significant eye irritation to cats and may also delay healing of the clear part of the eye (cornea) if it is damaged.

How Should It Be Given?
- Eye drops may be used every 2-6 hours depending on the condition that your veterinarian is treating.
- If you are giving more than one medication, you should allow 5 minutes between medications to allow the medication to work and to not be washed out by the next medication.
- Medication should be applied in the lower eyelid sac (conjunctival sac) without touching the tip of the dropper or tube to the eye as this will contaminate the medication. Do not touch the dropper or tube tip with your fingers as this will also contaminate the medication.

- The successful outcome of your animal's treatment with this medication depends upon your commitment and ability to administer it exactly as the veterinarian has prescribed. Please do not skip doses or stop giving the medication. If you have difficulty giving doses consult your veterinarian or pharmacist who can offer administration techniques or change the dosage form to a type of medication that may be more acceptable to you and your animal.
- If you miss a dose of this medication you should give it as soon as you remember it, but if it is within a few hours of the regularly scheduled dose, wait and give it at the regular time. Do not double a dose as this can be toxic to your pet.
- Some other drugs can interact with this medication so tell your veterinarian about any drugs or foods that you currently give your animal. Do not give new foods or medications without first asking your veterinarian.
- You should always wash your hands after applying this medication to your pet's eyes.
- **Dogs and Cats**: Trifluridine is not usually given to dogs, but is usually administered as a drop four to six times daily for cats. At the start of therapy, many veterinarians recommend using the drops every 2 hours for the first few days.
- **Horses**: Horses do not usually receive this medication.

What Other Information Is Important About This Medication?
- Trifluridine drops should be stored in a tight, light resistant, childproof container in the refrigerator away from all children and other household pets.
- Trifluridine may be very expensive.
- Your pet's eye should start to look better in 48 hours. If the eye looks the same or gets worse, you should contact your veterinarian for advice.

Triple Antibiotic (Neomycin, Bacitracin, Polymyxin) with Steroids Ophthalmic

AK Spore-HC®, Cortisporin®, Trioptic-S®, Maxitrol®, Dexacidin® and Gentocin Durafilm® are other names for these medications.

How Is This Medication Useful?

- Triple antibiotic solution (or ointment) with steroids is a combination of antibiotics and steroids that are used to treat inflammation of the eyes. Steroids should not be used if there is an infection present or if the eye has an ulcer.

Are There Conditions or Times When Its Use Might Cause More Harm Than Good?

- Some cats will have a fatal allergic (anaphylactic) reaction to the antibiotic combination of these drugs. It is not known which of the components is the cause of this fatal reaction. If your cat has swelling of the face or itching or looks like it is having difficulty breathing, you should take your cat to the closest veterinary clinic immediately.
- If your cat's eye looks worse after you start the medication, you should call your veterinarian.

What Side Effects Can Be Seen With Its Use?

- The medication may cause the eye to sting a bit when first put in the eye.
- Ointments will blur your animal's vision for a few minutes after administration. You should watch it for a short time to make sure it does not bump into things and injure itself.
- Side effects are unusual with this medication.

How Should It Be Given?

- Eye drops may be used every 2-6 hours and ointments every 8-12 depending on the condition that your veterinarian is treating.
- Solutions of this combination need to be shaken well before using.
- If you are giving more than one medication, you should allow 5 minutes between medications to allow the medication to work and to not be washed out by the next medication.

- Medication should be applied in the lower eyelid sac (conjunctival sac) without touching the tip of the dropper or tube to the eye as this will contaminate the medication. Do not touch the dropper or tube tip with your fingers as this will also contaminate the medication.
- The successful outcome of your animal's treatment with this medication depends upon your commitment and ability to administer it exactly as the veterinarian has prescribed. Please do not skip doses or stop giving the medication. If you have difficulty giving doses consult your veterinarian or pharmacist who can offer administration techniques or change the dosage form to a type of medication that may be more acceptable to you and your animal.
- If you miss a dose of this medication you should give it as soon as you remember it, but if it is within a few hours of the regularly scheduled dose, wait and give it at the regular time. Do not double a dose as this can be toxic to your pet.
- Some other drugs can interact with this medication so tell your veterinarian about any drugs or foods that you currently give your animal. Do not give new foods or medications without first asking your veterinarian.
- You should always wash your hands after applying this medication to your pet's eyes.
- **Dogs and Cats**: Triple antibiotic with steroids is usually administered as an ointment three to four times daily or as a solution four to six times daily. Steroids should not be used in the eyes of cats who are suffering from herpes keratitis as this may make the condition worse.
- **Horses**: Horses will usually receive triple antibiotic with steroids as an ointment once or twice daily. Steroids should never be used in an eye that has an ulcer.

What Other Information Is Important About This Medication?

- Triple antibiotic with steroids should be stored in a tight, light resistant, childproof container away from all children and other household pets.
- Your pet's eye should start to look better in 48 hours. If the eye looks the same or gets worse, you should contact your veterinarian for advice.

Triple Antibiotic (Neomycin, Bacitracin, Polymyxin) Ophthalmic

Neosporin® and triple antibiotic solution or ointment are other names for this medication.

How Is This Medication Useful?

- Triple antibiotic solution or ointment is a combination of antibiotics that are used to treat bacterial infections of the clear part of the eye (cornea) and the pink parts around the eyelids (conjunctiva). It is mostly used to treat animals with bacterial eye diseases or ulcers of the eye.

Are There Conditions or Times When Its Use Might Cause More Harm Than Good?

- Some cats will have a fatal allergic (anaphylactic) reaction to this combination of drugs. It is not known which of the components is the cause of this fatal reaction. If your cat has swelling of the face or itching or looks like it is having difficulty breathing, you should take your cat to the closest veterinary clinic immediately.
- If your cat's eye looks worse after you start the medication, you should call your veterinarian.

What Side Effects Can Be Seen With Its Use?

- The medication may cause the eye to sting a bit when first put in the eye.
- Ointments will blur your animal's vision for a few minutes after administration. You should watch it for a short time to make sure it does not bump into things and injure itself.
- Side effects are unusual with this medication.

How Should It Be Given?

- Eye drops may be used every 2-6 hours and ointments every 8-12 depending on the condition that your veterinarian is treating.
- If you are giving more than one medication, you should allow 5 minutes between medications to allow the medication to work and to not be washed out by the next medication. If you are placing medications through the catheter system, you should push some air, not liquid, through the tubing between drugs to push the drops to the eye.
- Medication should be applied in the lower eyelid sac (conjunctival sac) without touching the tip of the dropper or tube to the eye as this will contaminate the medication. Do not touch the dropper or tube tip with your fingers as this will also contaminate the medication.

- The successful outcome of your animal's treatment with this medication depends upon your commitment and ability to administer it exactly as the veterinarian has prescribed. Please do not skip doses or stop giving the medication. If you have difficulty giving doses consult your veterinarian or pharmacist who can offer administration techniques or change the dosage form to a type of medication that may be more acceptable to you and your animal.
- If you miss a dose of this medication you should give it as soon as you remember it, but if it is within a few hours of the regularly scheduled dose, wait and give it at the regular time. Do not double a dose as this can be toxic to your pet.
- Some other drugs can interact with this medication so tell your veterinarian about any drugs or foods that you currently give your animal. Do not give new foods or medications without first asking your veterinarian.
- You should always wash your hands after applying this medication to your pet's eyes.
- **Dogs and Cats**: Triple antibiotic is usually administered as an ointment three to four times daily or as a solution four to six times daily.
- **Horses**: Horses will usually receive triple antibiotic solution as a solution administered through an eye catheter (subpalpebral lavage system) every one to four hours or as an ointment once or twice daily.

What Other Information Is Important About This Medication?

- Triple antibiotic solution should be stored in a tight, light resistant, childproof container away from all children and other household pets.
- Your pet's eye should start to look better in 48 hours. If the eye looks the same or gets worse, you should contact your veterinarian for advice.

Tropicamide Ophthalmic

Mydriacyl® is another name for this medication.

How Is This Medication Useful?

- Tropicamide is used in the eye to dilate the pupil. This effect is useful in reducing pain after cataract surgery or eye injury and is also useful in treating glaucoma.

Are There Conditions or Times When Its Use Might Cause More Harm Than Good?

- Condition may worsen with tropicamide use in dogs with primary glaucoma.
- Using tropicamide in the eye more frequently than prescribed can result in serious problems such as colic in horses and a dangerous increase in body temperature in other animals.
- Tropicamide toxicity may also cause some changes in heart rate and rhythm and may cause your pet to be unable to urinate.
- If your animal has any of the above conditions, talk to your veterinarian about the potential risks of using the medication versus the benefits that it might have.

What Side Effects Can Be Seen With Its Use?

- Because tropicamide dilates the pupil, animals will be very sensitive to sunlight and should be kept out of bright light while receiving this drug.
- Most animals will salivate when tropicamide drops get into their mouth.
- Too much tropicamide can result in dry mouth, constipation and vomiting.

How Should It Be Given?

- The successful outcome of your animal's treatment with this medication depends upon your commitment and ability to administer it exactly as the veterinarian has prescribed. Please do not skip doses or stop giving the medication. If you have difficulty giving doses consult your veterinarian or pharmacist who can offer administration techniques or change the dosage form to a type of medication that may be more acceptable to you and your animal.

- If you miss a dose of this medication you should give it as soon as you remember it, but if it is within a few hours of the regularly scheduled dose, wait and give it at the regular time. Do not double a dose as this can be toxic to your pet.
- Some other drugs can interact with this medication so tell your veterinarian about any drugs or foods that you currently give your animal. Do not give new foods or medications without first asking your veterinarian.
- You should always wash your hands after applying this medication to your pet's eyes as it can get into your eyes and cause dilation of the pupil.
- **Dogs and Cats**: Tropicamide is usually administered three times daily after cataract surgery in dogs and cats.
- **Horses**: Horses usually receive atropine sulfate instead of tropicamide.

What Other Information Is Important About This Medication?

- Tropicamide should be stored in a tight, light resistant, childproof container away from all children and other household pets.
- Hands should be washed after application as you may get tropicamide in your own eye and cause the pupil to dilate (get bigger) making it difficult to see or painful to be in bright sunlight.

Applying Transdermal Medications to Cats

You should store this medication at room temperature away from heat and light and out of the reach of children. This package is not child-proof.

Directions:

1. Your pharmacist will have provided you with gloves or glove finger tips with the transdermal medication. Place a glove tip on both thumb and index finger.

2. Use a damp paper towel or cotton ball to clean the inside of the cat's ear. Do not attempt to clean the cat's ear canals, it is not necessary or desirable to do so.

3. Remove the tip from one syringe and squirt entire contents (or the amount for the correct dose for your cat) on tip of gloved index finger.

4. Apply to inside of cat's ear (pinna) with index finger and use thumb and finger to massage into ear until completely absorbed. Do not touch the drug with your bare hands.

5. Do not get any drug into the canals (horizontal or vertical) of the ears.

6. Using ungloved hand, turn on faucet and rinse gloved fingertips carefully under running water.

7. Fling tips off fingers into sink (being careful not to invert glove tip).

8. Pick up and thoroughly dry with disposable paper towel.

9. Return clean, dry glove tips to zip lock bag for next use.

VETERINARY DRUG HANDBOOK-Client Information Edition
Permission to photocopy for individual clients granted by Gigi Davidson and Donald C. Plumb © 2003

Giving Your Cat Oral Medications

1. Relax. If your cat senses that you are upset or anxious, it will be, too! Make sure you have all the medication ready to give (tablets and capsules loose, liquids drawn up in oral syringes) before you catch the cat. Coating the tablet with butter or some other tasty substance such as tuna or anchovy paste will lubricate the medication and give it a desirable taste. This may make it easier to medicate reluctant cats. It may also be helpful to have another person standing ready in case you need assistance.

2. Place your cat on a slippery, slick surface such as a table or counter top. This will keep it from getting a grip with its claws and running away. Sometimes it may be helpful to wrap your cat in a towel or blanket, so that its feet will be restrained. It is always useful to trim your cat's claws before attempting medication therapy.

3. With one hand, calmly grasp the top of the cat's head. The tips of your thumb and index finger should be positioned at opposite corners of the mouth on the cat's upper lip.

4. Gently tilt the cat's head back so that its chin is facing upward.

5. Holding the pill between the thumb and index finger of the other hand, place downward pressure with your middle finger on the front of the cat's lower jaw. This pressure, together with tilting the cat's head, will cause the cat to open its mouth. If it does not, then use your middle finger to gently pry open the lower jaw.

6. Quickly drop or slide the pill as far back in the mouth or throat as possible. Once the pill is positioned in the back of the mouth, it is unlikely that the cat will spit it out!

7. If you are giving liquid, do not tilt your cat's chin up. Instead, introduce the liquid filled syringe just past the lower teeth and slowly squirt small amounts into the mouth. Pause between amounts to allow your cat to swallow all the liquid.

8. Studies have shown that tablets and capsules do not get stuck between the throat and the stomach if a small amount of water (6ml or about 1 teaspoonful) is given immediately after giving the medication. This can be done via a medicine dropper or syringe. If your cat is calm and willing, offering it a small saucer with a tablespoonful or milk or tuna juice will make sure that the medication gets washed down to the stomach. Check with your veterinarian or pharmacist to see what foods and liquids are compatible with the medication you are giving.

9. If you think the cat has not swallowed the medication, blowing in its face or gently rubbing its throat may stimulate the cat to swallow.

10. Excessive salivation may be seen in some cats after receiving medications. This is not harmful and will subside once the cat relaxes.

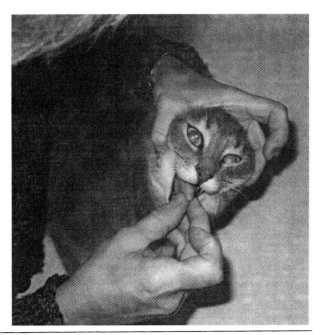

Giving Your Dog Oral Medications

1. Get all the drugs ready and lay them out next to where you are going to give them. This includes shaking up oral liquids and drawing the correct dose into the syringe. Tablets and capsules may be wrapped in a small piece of meat or bread that your dog likes.

2. Relax! Ask your dog to come to you in a relaxed, happy voice. If your dog senses that you are upset or anxious, it will be, too!

3. Take your dog to a corner, and face his rear end into the corner so he cannot back away from you.

4. Using your free hand, calmly grasp your dog's muzzle from above with your fingers on one side and thumb on the other with tips at corner of your dog's mouth.

5. Squeeze behind the upper canine teeth ("fangs") and gently tilt its head back until his chin is pointing upwards. His lower jaw should automatically open a little bit. Use one of the other fingers of your other hand to open the right hand to open the lower jaw further by pushing on the bottom teeth with one of your fingers to pry it open.

6. Quickly place the pill as far back in your dog's mouth as possible, preferably on the back of the tongue. Do not place your hand too far in, however, or your dog may choke and gag.

7. If you are giving liquid medication, do not raise your pet's chin up, but instead, introduce the tip of the syringe just past the lower teeth and squirt small amounts into your dog's mouth. Pause between squirts to allow him to swallow the medication without gagging or choking.

8. Gently lower his head and close your dog's mouth by wrapping your fingers around its muzzle. Gently rubbing or blowing on your dog's nose may help stimulate him to swallow.

9. Give your dog plenty of praise, and possibly a treat. This will make next time easier. And remember, the quicker you can give the medication, the easier it is on both of you.

10. The most important part of drug therapy is getting all of the drug that your veterinarian has prescribed into your dog for the entire time that he has prescribed therapy. If you have difficulty getting all of the medication into your dog, call your veterinarian for advice or assistance.

VETERINARY DRUG HANDBOOK-Client Information Edition
Permission to photocopy for individual clients granted by Gigi Davidson and Donald C. Plumb © 2003

Giving Your Horse Oral Medications

1. Giving medication to a horse is always a challenge. Ideally, you can give the medication as a flavored powder that can be mixed in the feed so the horse will eat the medication without knowing it. If you give medication this way, make sure you check the bottom of the feed bucket about 30 minutes after the horse has finished eating to ensure that all medication has been swallowed.

2. Many drugs, however, must be given directly in the horse's mouth. Before you bring the horse up to be treated, make sure that you have adequately prepared all the doses of medication. This means crushing any tablets into a powder and mixing with molasses or some other favorite flavor in a syringe, or drawing up liquids into a dosing syringe, or dialing the appropriate dose on a paste syringe and having it ready to squirt into the horse's mouth. Ask your veterinarian or pharmacist before mixing any medications with food or flavors to make sure that they won't inhibit the drug's effect.

3. Securely cross tie the horse or have a strong person hold the horse with a halter and lead rope. It is always good to have someone there to help you in case you have difficulty.

4. If you are giving large tablets (boluses), you may need a balling gun to give the medication. A balling gun is a plunger device that holds the bolus at the end of the plunger until placed in the back of the horse's mouth where the bolus can then be popped into the horse's mouth. Be sure that the horse actually swallows the bolus and does not spit it out.

5. If you are giving medication in a syringe, place the tip of the syringe in the corner of your horse's mouth. Elevate the horse's head slightly by lifting the halter or lead line. Wiggle the syringe tip back and forth against the tongue to stimulate movement of the tongue. When the tongue starts moving, start squirting paste onto the tongue and gums. The contents of the syringe will stick to the tongue and gums and ensure that the horse will eventually swallow the medication.

6. Some drugs may be irritating to the mouth and gums, so your veterinarian may want you to rinse your horse's mouth out with water after giving these medications.

7. The most important part of drug therapy is getting all of the drug that your veterinarian has prescribed into your horse for the entire time that he has prescribed therapy. If you have difficulty getting all of the medication into your horse, call your veterinarian for advice or assistance.

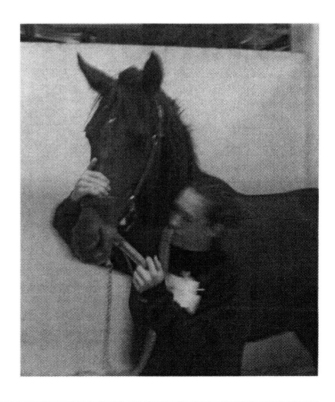

How To Administer Eye Medications To Your Pet

1. Gather up all the eye medications that you are going to administer to your pet.

2. It is very important that once finished that you replace the top that goes with its original container. While using the medication, either leave the tops in a place where you won't confuse them with one another or preferably, open and use each medication and then immediately replace the container top. The second option works best when you have a helper available.

3. Call or catch your pet and calmly bring them to the area where you plan to give the drops. Relax! If you are anxious or nervous, your pet will be, too.

4. Firmly grasp the pet under the chin and lift its chin and eyes towards the ceiling. Position your other hand over the pet's head bringing the dropper bottle or ointment tube just above the eyes.

If you are giving eye drops:

5. Pull the lower eyelid down slightly.

6. Squeeze the eye drops into the inner corner of eye taking care not to touch the dropper to the eye surface.

7. Continue to hold the head back for a moment or two while the drops disperse over the whole eye surface.

8. Do not touch the eye itself with the dropper.

If you are giving eye ointment:

5. Be sure that the tip of the tube is pointed away from your pet's eye so that if they jerk, the tube tip will not injure the eye.

6. Pull the lower eyelid down slightly.

7. Squeeze a thin strip of the ointment along the inner side of the lower eyelid.

8. Have your pet blink and gently hold its eyelid shut; gently massage the closed eyelid to help disperse the ointment

9. Your pet's vision will be blurry for a few minutes while the ointment melts. Watch your pet to make sure that it does not bump into things while its vision is blurred.

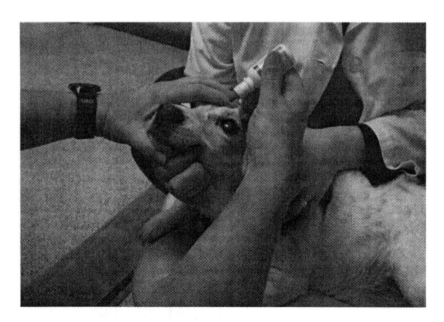

VETERINARY DRUG HANDBOOK-Client Information Edition
Permission to photocopy for individual clients granted by Gigi Davidson and Donald C. Plumb © 2003

If Your Pet Gets Into Poison

If your pet gets into a drug or poison, you should call your veterinarian immediately. There are six important questions you should do your best to know the answers to before you call. Write down the information below so you can tell your veterinarian.

1. What did the pet get into? Write down the name of the product and the active ingredients if they are listed.

2. How much did the pet get into?

3. Did the animal swallow it or get it in their eyes or on their skin?

4. How long ago was it?

5. How is your pet acting?

6. How long has it been acting that way?

If the pet has swallowed a potential poison, your veterinarian may want you to try some things at home before the animal is brought into the clinic.

- If your veterinarian tells you it is okay to make your pet vomit (*i.e.*, not unconscious, not seizuring (convulsions), not drowsy, able to gag, and the poison is not a corrosive toxin or petroleum distillate) then you can induce vomiting.

- Save the vomit by placing in a zip-loc bag or other clean and sealable container. If vomiting could worsen the poison effects, your veterinarian may want you to administer milk or water to dilute the poison.

- Drugs that cause vomiting available in most homes include:
  - Syrup of ipecac 7%; your veterinarian will tell you how much to give
  - Hydrogen peroxide 3%: 1 teaspoonful orally

- If your animal does not vomit after giving these, do not give them again unless your veterinarian tells you to.

- If the animal has gotten the poison in its eyes or on its skin, you should immediately wash the animal with lots of warm water or flush the eyes with a preservative free contact lens rinsing solution.

- If the animal is seizuring (convulsing), you should to try to help protect the animal from injuring itself by removing lamps, tables, chairs and other objects that it could hurt itself on. Do not put your hands in or near the animal's mouth. Your pet will not swallow its tongue during the seizure, but it may unintentionally bite you if you put your hands in its mouth.

- You should get your pet to a veterinary clinic as soon as possible.

- Bring whatever container is available of the poison and any vomit that was produced.

Index

2-aminosulphonic acid, 137

Acetaminophen, 1
Acetazolamide, 2
Actigall®, 145
Acular®, 157
AK Spore-HC®, 165
Albuterol, 4
Aldactone®, 133
Aller-Chlor®, 36
Allopurinol, 5
Alpha tocopherol, 146
Altrenogest, 6
Amicar®, 7
Aminocaproic acid, 7
Aminoglycoside opth., 148
Aminophylline, 8
Amitriptyline, 9
Amlodipine, 10
Ammonium chloride, 11
Amoxicillin, 12
Amoxicillin/Clavulanate, 13
Amoxil®, 12
Amoxitabs®, 12
Amphicol®, 35
Anafranil®, 43
Anipryl®, 131
Antihist-1®, 40
Antirobe®, 42
APAP, 1
Apresoline®, 73
Ascorbic acid, 14
Aspirin, 15
Atarax®, 75
Atenolol, 16
Atrophate®, 149
Atropine sulfate ophthalmic, 149
Augmentin®, 13
Azathioprine, 17
Azulfidine®, 136

Baclofen, 18
Bactrim®, 142
Banamine®, 68
Baytril®, 60
Bemacol®, 150
Benadryl®, 56
Benazepril, 19
Betapace®, 132
Bethanechol, 20
Biocef®, 33
Biosol®, 104
Bisacodyl, 21
Bismukote®, 22
Bismusal®, 22
Bismuth subsalicylate, 22
Brethine®, 138
Bricanyl®, 138

Bromides, 23
Bromocriptine, 24
Buprenex®, 25
Buprenorphine, 25
Buspar®, 26
Buspirone, 26
Butatab®, 116
Butazolidin®, 116
Bute, 116
Butorphanol, 27

Capoten®, 28
Captopril, 28
Carafate®, 135
Cardizem®, 55
Cardoxin®, 54
Carnitine, 29
Carprofen, 30
Cefa-Drops®, 31
Cefadroxil, 31
Cefa-Tabs®, 31
Cefixime, 32
Cephalexin, 33
Cephulac®, 86
Chibroxin®, 162
Chlorambucil, 34
Chloramphenicol, 35, 150
Chloramphenicol ophth., 150
Chlorbiotic®, 150
Chloricol®, 150
Chloromycetin®, 35
Chlorpheniramine, 36
Chlorpromazine, 37
Chlortrimeton®, 36
Chronulac®, 86
Ciloxan®, 162
Cimetidine, 38
Ciprofloxacin ophth., 162
Cisapride, 39
Clavamox®, 13
Clavulanate, 13
Clavulanate/Amoxicillin, 13
Clemastine, 40
Clenbuterol, 41
Cleocin®, 42
Clindamycin, 42
Clomicalm®, 43
Clomipramine, 43
Codeine, 44
Corrective Mixture®, 22
Cortef®, 123
Corticosteroid ophth., 151
Corticosteroids, 151
Cortisporin®, 165
Coumadin®, 147
Cutter Tape Tabs®, 122
Cyclophosphamide, 45
Cyclosporine ophth., 152
Cyclosporine, 46

Cyproheptadine, 47
Cytomel®, 89
Cytotec®, 100
Cytoxan®, 45

Dalteparin, 48
d-carnitine, 29
DDAVP®, 50
Decadron®, 151
Depo-Medrol®, 95
Deracoxib, 49
Deramaxx®, 49
DES, 53
Desmopressin, 50
Dexacidin®, 165
Diamox®, 2
Diazepam, 51
Diazoxide, 52
Dibenzyline®, 115
Diethylstilbestero, 53
Diflucan®, 66
Digoxin, 54
Dilacor®, 55
Diltiazem, 55
Diphenhydramine, 56
Disal®, 70
Ditropan®, 109
Dorzolamide ophth., 153
Doxepin, 57
Doxycycline, 58
Droncit®, 122
Drontal Plus®, 122
Drontal®, 122
Dulcolax®, 21
Duragesic®, 65
Duricef®, 31
Duricol®, 35

Econopred®, 151
EES®, 61
Elavil®, 9
Eldepryl®, 131
E-Mycin®, 61
Enacard®, 59
Enalapril, 59
Enrofloxacin, 60
Equimectrin®, 81
Eqvalan®, 81
Erygel®, 61
Erythrocin®, 61
Erythromycin, 61
Etodolac, 62
Etogesic®, 62

Famotidine, 63
Feldene®, 121
Fenbendazole, 64
Fentanyl, 65
Flagyl®, 98

Florinef®, 67
Fluconazole, 66
Fludrocortisone, 67
Flunixin, 68
Fluoxetine, 69
Flurbiprofen ophth., 154
Fragmin®, 48
Fulvicin®, 72
Furosemide, 70

Garamycin®, 148
Gastrogard®, 105
Gengraf®, 46
Gentocin Durafilm®, 165
Gentocin®, 148
Glipizide, 71
Glucotrol®, 71
Grifulvin®, 72
Grisactin®, 72
Griseofulvin, 72
Gris-PEG®, 72

Heartgard®, 81
Humilin®, 77
Hycodan®, 74
Hydralazine, 73
Hydrocodone, 74
Hydroxyzine, 75

Idoxuridine ophth., 155
Iletin®, 77
Imipramine, 76
Imuran®, 17
Inderal®, 126
Insulin, 77
Interceptor®, 99
Interferon, 79
Intron®, 79
Itraconazole, 80
Itraconazole ophth., 156
Ivermectin, 81
Ivomec®, 81

KBr, 23
K-Caps, 119
Keflex®, 33
Keftab®, 33
Ketoconazole, 83
Ketofen®, 85
Ketoprofen, 85
Ketorolac ophth., 157

Lactulose, 86
Lanoxin®, 54
Lasix®, 70
Latanaprost ophth., 158
L-carnitine, 29
L-deprenyl, 131
Leukeran®, 34
Levocarnitine, 29
Levothyroxine, 87
Lincocin®, 88
Lincomycin, 88
Lioresal®, 18
Liothyronine, 89

Lodine®, 62
Lotensin®, 19
L-thyroxine, 87
Lufenuron, 90
Luminal®, 114
Lysodren®, 101

Marbofloxacin, 91
Maxitrol®, 165
Medrol®, 95
Meloxicam, 92
Mephyton, 119
Mestinon®, 128
Metacam®, 92
Methapred®, 95
Methimazole, 93
Methocarbamol, 94
Methylprednisolone, 95
Metoclopramide, 97
Metrogel®, 98
Metronidazole, 98
Miconazole ophth., 159
Milbemycin, 99
Misoprostol, 100
Mitotane, 101
Mobic®, 92
Modane®, 21
Monistat®, 159
Morphine, 103
Mydriacyl®, 167

Natacyn®, 160
Natamycin ophth., 160
Nemex®, 127
Neomycin sulfate, 104
Neoral®, 46
Neosporin®, 166
Nexium®, 105
Nizoral®, 83
Norfloxacin ophth., 162
Norvasc®, 10
Novolin®, 77

o,p-DDD, 101
Ocufen®, 154
Ocuflox®, 162
Ofloxacin ophth., 162
Omeprazole, 105
Ondansetron, 106
Optimune®, 152
Orbax®, 107
Orbifloxacin, 107
Orudis®, 85
Oxazepam, 108
Oxybutynin, 109
Oxytetracycline ophth., 161

Panacur®, 64
Pancrelipase, 110
Pancrezyme®, 110
Panmycin®, 139
Paracetamol, 1
Parlodel®, 24
Paroxetine, 111
Paxil®, 111

Pentoxifylline, 112
Pepcid®, 63
Pepto Bismol®, 22
Pergolide, 113
Periactin®, 47
Permax®, 113
Phenobarbital, 114
Phenobarbitone, 114
Phenoxybenzamine, 115
Phenylbutazone, 116
Phenylbute®, 116
Phenylpropanolamine, 118
Phenylzone®, 116
Phytonadione, 119
Pipa-Tabs®, 120
Piperazine, 120
Piroxicam, 121
Potassium bromide, 23
Praziquantel, 122
Pred Forte®, 151
Prednisolone, 141
Prednisolone, 123
Prednisone, 123
Prednis-tab®, 123
Prelone®, 123
Prilosec®, 105
Probanthine®, 125
Proglycem®, 52
Program®, 90
Proin®, 118
Propadrine®, 118
Propantheline, 125
Propranolol, 126
Propulsid®, 39
Protostat®, 98
Proventil®, 4
Prozac®, 69
Pyrantel, 127
Pyridostigmine, 128

Ranitidine, 129
Reglan®, 97
Regumate®, 6
Rifadin®, 130
Rifampin, 130
Rimactane®, 130
Rimadyl®, 30
Robaxin®, 94
Roferon-A®, 79

Safe-Guard®, 64
Salix®, 70
Sandimmune®, 46
Selegilene, 131
Septra®, 142
Serax®, 108
Sinequan®, 57
Slo-bid®, 140
Slo-Phyllin®, 140
Slo-phylline®, 8
Sodium bromide, 23
Solfoton®, 114
Soloxine®, 87
Solu-Delta-Cortef®, 123

Solu-Medrol®, 95
Sotalol, 132
Spironolactone, 133
Sporanox®, 80
Sporonox®, 156
Stadol®, 27
Stanozolol, 134
Stilphostrol®, 53
Stoxil®, 155
Strongid-T®, 127
Sucralfate, 135
Sulfasalazine, 136
Sumycin®, 139
Suprax®, 32
Synthroid®, 87

Tagamet®, 38
Tapazole®, 93
Taurine, 137
Tavist®, 40
Temaril-P®, 141
Tenormin®, 16
Terbutaline, 138
Terramycin®, 161
Tetracycline, 139
Theobid®, 140
Theolair®, 140
Theophylline, 140
Thorazine®, 37
Thyro-Form®, 87
Thyro-L®, 87
Thyro-Tabs®, 87
Timolol ophth., 163
Timoptic®, 163
Tobrex®, 148
Tofranil®, 76
Torbugesic®, 27
Torbutrol®, 27
Torpex®, 4
Trental®, 112
Tribrissen®, 142
Trifluridine ophth., 164
Trimeprazine, 141
Trimethoprim/Sulfa, 142
Trimox®, 12
Trioptic-S®, 165
Triple antibiotic ophth., 166
Triple antibiotic solution w/
    steroids ophth., 165
Tropicamide ophth., 167
Trusopt®, 153
Tucoprim®, 142
Tussigon®, 74
Tylan®, 144
Tylenol®, 1
Tylosin, 144

Ultramectrin®, 81
Urecholine®, 20
Uroeze®, 11
Ursodiol, 145

Valium®, 51

Valproic acid, 29
Vasotec®, 59
Veda-K1, 119
Ventipulmin®, 41
Veta-K1, 119
Vibramycin®, 58
Viceton®, 35
Viokase®, 110
Viroptic®, 164
Vistaril®, 75
Vitamin Bt, 29
Vitamin C, 14
Vitamin E, 146

Warfarin, 147
Winstrol®, 134
Wymox®, 12

Xalatan®, 158

Zantac®, 129
Zeniquin®, 91
Zimectrin®, 81
Zofran®, 106
Zyloprim®, 5

LaVergne, TN USA
09 March 2010
175325LV00001B/3/A